Copyright

MCQ in Basic Pharmacology: Comprehensive Self-Assessment for Medical, Nursing Students, and Healthcare Professionals

The multiple-choice questions and explanations in this book are designed to assist learning, self-assessment, and examination preparation. They should not be considered a substitute for professional medical education, clinical training, or independent clinical judgment.

Neither the author nor the publisher shall be liable for any loss, injury, or damage resulting from the use of the information contained in this publication.

First Edition: 2026

Printed in the United States of America

Author: Emil Zaki

ISBN: Assigned by Amazon KDP or enter your own ISBN here.

Preface

Pharmacology is one of the most essential and challenging subjects in the education of healthcare professionals. A thorough understanding of drugs, their mechanisms of action, therapeutic uses, adverse effects, contraindications, and interactions is fundamental to safe and effective patient care. Whether preparing for academic examinations, licensing assessments, or daily clinical practice, a strong foundation in pharmacology is indispensable.

MCQ in Basic Pharmacology: Comprehensive Self-Assessment for Medical, Nursing Students, and Healthcare Professionals has been developed to provide an organized and practical resource for learners seeking to master the principles and clinical applications of pharmacology. The book contains carefully designed multiple-choice questions covering the major areas of basic and clinical pharmacology, ranging from general pharmacological principles and pharmacokinetics to organ-system pharmacology, antimicrobial agents, anticancer drugs, toxicology, and medication safety.

The questions are structured to reinforce core concepts while encouraging analytical thinking and clinical reasoning. Many questions are presented in an examination style similar to those encountered in university examinations, nursing examinations, licensing assessments, and professional certification tests. Each question is followed by a detailed explanation that not only identifies the correct answer but also explains the reasoning behind it, highlights important clinical points, and clarifies why the alternative options are incorrect. This approach transforms every question into an effective learning opportunity rather than simply a testing exercise.

This book is intended for:

- Medical students preparing for professional examinations.
- Nursing students studying pharmacology and therapeutics.
- Pharmacy and allied health students seeking comprehensive review.
- Physician assistants and other healthcare trainees.
- Practicing physicians, nurses, pharmacists, and healthcare professionals wishing to refresh and update their pharmacological knowledge.
- Candidates preparing for mock examinations, licensing examinations, and postgraduate entrance assessments.

To maximize the benefit of this book, readers are encouraged to answer each question independently before consulting the explanation. Revisiting incorrectly answered questions and reviewing the accompanying explanations will strengthen understanding and improve long-term retention of essential pharmacological concepts.

While every effort has been made to ensure the accuracy and relevance of the material presented, pharmacology is a rapidly evolving discipline. New medications, revised clinical guidelines, and updated recommendations continue to emerge. Therefore, readers are encouraged to consult current clinical guidelines, official prescribing information, and institutional protocols when making therapeutic decisions in clinical practice. This book is intended as an educational resource and should not replace professional clinical judgment or evidence-based medical guidance.

It is my sincere hope that this book will serve as a valuable companion throughout your educational journey and professional career, helping you build confidence, improve examination performance, and enhance your ability to provide safe, effective, and evidence-based patient care.

I wish you every success in your studies, examinations, and future practice.

Emil Zaki

How to Use This Book

Welcome to MCQ in Basic Pharmacology: Comprehensive Self-Assessment for Medical, Nursing Students, and Healthcare Professionals. This book has been carefully designed to help you build a strong foundation in pharmacology, evaluate your understanding, and prepare effectively for examinations and clinical practice.

To gain the greatest benefit from this book, consider the following approach:

1. Assess Your Knowledge

Begin each section by answering the multiple-choice questions without referring to textbooks or notes. This will help you identify your strengths and the topics that require additional review.

2. Read Every Explanation

Each question is accompanied by a detailed explanation. Even if you answer correctly, read the explanation to reinforce key concepts, understand the underlying pharmacological principles, and recognize important clinical applications.

3. Learn from Incorrect Answers

The explanations clarify why the correct answer is the best choice and why the other options are incorrect. Reviewing these distinctions will strengthen your clinical reasoning and improve your performance on future examinations.

4. Study One Topic at a Time

The book is organized into major pharmacology topics. Focus on one section at a time before moving to the next. Mastering each topic individually promotes better understanding and long-term retention.

5. Simulate Examination Conditions

For effective exam preparation, answer a group of questions under timed conditions without using external resources. This practice improves time management, confidence, and test-taking skills.

6. Review Regularly

Repetition is essential for retaining pharmacological knowledge. Revisit questions you previously answered incorrectly and periodically review completed sections to reinforce learning.

7. Apply Knowledge to Clinical Practice

Whenever possible, relate the pharmacological principles to real or simulated clinical scenarios. Understanding how medications are selected, administered, monitored, and managed in patient care enhances both examination performance and professional competence.

8. Use the Comprehensive Mock Examination

After completing all sections, take the final comprehensive mock examination as a self-assessment. This examination is intended to simulate the breadth and style of questions commonly encountered in university examinations, licensing assessments, and professional certification tests.

9. Keep Current with Clinical Practice

Pharmacology is a rapidly evolving field. While this book provides a solid foundation, readers should consult current clinical guidelines, official prescribing information, and institutional protocols for the most up-to-date recommendations.

Who Will Benefit from This Book?

This book is suitable for:

Medical students

Nursing students

Pharmacy students

Physician assistant students

Allied health students

Medical interns and residents

Registered nurses

Pharmacists

Physicians and other healthcare professionals seeking a comprehensive review of pharmacology

Study Tips for Success

- Study consistently rather than cramming before examinations.
- Focus on understanding drug mechanisms instead of memorizing isolated facts.
- Pay special attention to drug indications, contraindications, adverse effects, drug interactions, and major clinical precautions.
- Review high-yield topics repeatedly.
- Use incorrect answers as opportunities to strengthen your understanding.
- Complete the comprehensive mock examination before your final examination or licensing test.

With consistent study and active practice, this book will help you strengthen your pharmacological knowledge, improve your examination performance, and enhance your confidence in making safe, evidence-based medication decisions in clinical practice.

We wish you every success in your studies, examinations, and professional career.

Table of Contents

Part I – General Principles of Pharmacology

Part I – General Principles of Pharmacology

Introduction

General Principles of Pharmacology form the foundation upon which all pharmacological knowledge is built. Before studying individual drugs and their clinical applications, it is essential to understand how medications interact with the human body, how the body processes drugs, and the principles that guide their safe and effective use.

This section introduces the fundamental concepts of pharmacology that every medical, nursing, pharmacy, and allied health student should master. These principles are frequently tested in undergraduate examinations, licensing examinations, and professional certification assessments because they underpin rational prescribing and safe patient care.

The multiple-choice questions in this section are designed to assess your understanding of the core concepts that govern drug therapy. Topics include drug nomenclature and classification, sources of drugs, mechanisms of drug action, receptor pharmacology, agonists and antagonists, dose–response relationships, therapeutic index, drug safety, adverse drug reactions, and the principles of evidence- based pharmacotherapy.

A thorough understanding of these concepts will enable you to:

- Explain how drugs produce their therapeutic and adverse effects.
- Understand the relationship between drug dose and clinical response.
- Differentiate between potency, efficacy, and therapeutic effectiveness.
- Recognize factors that influence drug safety and toxicity.
- Apply pharmacological principles to rational prescribing and medication management .
- Interpret pharmacological information encountered in clinical practice and medical literature.

The questions range from fundamental knowledge to clinical application, encouraging both recall and critical thinking. Carefully review the explanations provided after each question, as they reinforce key concepts, clarify common misconceptions, and highlight important examination points.

Learning Objectives

After completing this section, you should be able to:

- Define pharmacology and its major branches.
- Classify drugs according to their source, chemical structure, mechanism of action, and therapeutic use.
- Describe the different types of drug receptors and mechanisms of drug action. Distinguish between agonists, partial agonists, inverse agonists, and antagonists. Explain receptor affinity, efficacy, potency, and selectivity.
- Interpret dose–response curves and therapeutic index.
- Identify factors affecting drug response, including patient-related variables. Recognize common adverse drug reactions and medication errors.
- Understand the principles of safe and rational drug prescribing.
- Apply evidence-based principles when selecting and evaluating drug therapy.

Topics Covered

1.Definition and Scope of Pharmacology
2.Branches of Pharmacology
3.Drug Nomenclature
4.Drug Classification
5.Sources of Drugs
6.Routes of Drug Administration
7.Drug Receptors
8.Mechanisms of Drug Action
9.Agonists and Antagonists
10.Dose–Response Relationships
11.Potency and Efficacy
12.Therapeutic Index
13.Drug Selectivity
14.Adverse Drug Reactions
15.Drug Safety
16.Medication Errors
17.Essential Medicines
18.Generic and Brand-Name Drugs
19.Rational Drug Use
20.Principles of Evidence-Based Pharmacotherapy

Number of Questions: 100

Difficulty Level: Beginner to Intermediate

Mastering the general principles presented in this section will provide the essential knowledge needed to understand the pharmacology of every drug class discussed in the chapters that follow and will establish a strong foundation for success in examinations and clinical practice.

Definition and Scope of Pharmacology

Definition of Pharmacology

Pharmacology is the branch of biomedical science that studies drugs and their interactions with living organisms. It encompasses the origin, chemical properties, mechanisms of action, therapeutic uses, adverse effects, metabolism, excretion, and safe administration of medications.

A drug is any chemical substance that, when administered to a living organism, produces a biological effect by modifying physiological functions or disease processes. Drugs are used to prevent, diagnose, treat, or relieve the symptoms of disease and to improve the quality of life.

Pharmacology provides the scientific foundation for the rational and safe use of medications in clinical practice. It bridges the gap between basic medical sciences and patient care, enabling healthcare professionals to select the most appropriate medication, determine the correct dosage, minimize adverse effects, and optimize therapeutic outcomes.

Scope of Pharmacology

Thescope of pharmacology extends from the discovery of new drugs in the

laboratory to their safe and effective use in patients. It includes the study of how drugs act on the body, how the body handles drugs, and how medications are used to prevent and treat disease.

Major areas within pharmacology include:

1. Pharmacokinetics

The study of what the body does to the drug, including:

- Absorption
- Distribution
- Metabolism
- Excretion (ADME)

Understanding pharmacokinetics helps determine the appropriate dose, route of administration, dosing interval, and duration of therapy.

2. Pharmacodynamics

The study of what the drug does to the body, including:

- Mechanism of action
- Drug receptors
- Therapeutic effects
- Adverse effects
- Dose–response relationships

3. Clinical Pharmacology

Clinical pharmacology focuses on the safe and effective use of drugs in human patients. It emphasizes:

Rational prescribing

Therapeutic drug monitoring

Drug interactions

Individualized therapy

Evidence-based medicine

4. Toxicology

Toxicology is the study of the harmful effects of drugs, chemicals, and poisons.

It includes:

- Drug overdose
- Poisoning
- Adverse drug reactions
- Antidotes
- Prevention and management of toxicity

5. Chemotherapy

Chemotherapy refers to the use of chemical agents to treat infectious diseases and cancer.

Examples include:

Antibiotics

Antiviral drugs

Antifungal agents

Antiparasitic drugs

Anticancer medications

6. Pharmacogenomics

Pharmacogenomics examines how genetic variations influence an individual's response to medications.

Its goals include:

- Personalized medicine Improved drug efficacy
- Reduced adverse drug reactions Individualized drug

7. Pharmacoepidemiology

This field studies the use and effects of drugs in large populations.

Applications include:

- Drug safety surveillance
- Monitoring adverse drug reactions
- Evaluating prescribing patterns
- Public health research

8. Pharmacovigilance

Pharmacovigilance is the science of detecting, assessing, understanding, and preventing adverse effects or other drug-related problems after medications have been marketed.

Importance of Pharmacology

A sound understanding of pharmacology enables healthcare professionals to:

- Select the most appropriate medication for each patient.
- Prescribe drugs safely and effectively.
- Prevent medication errors.
- Recognize and manage adverse drug reactions.
- Identify important drug interactions.
- Adjust drug therapy for patients with renal or hepatic impairment.
- Improve patient outcomes through evidence-based prescribing.

Learning Outcomes

After studying this topic, you should be able to:

- Define pharmacology.
- Explain the role of pharmacology in healthcare.
- Describe the major branches of pharmacology.
- Differentiate between pharmacokinetics and pharmacodynamics.
- Explain the importance of toxicology, clinical pharmacology, and pharmacovigilance.
- Recognize the contribution of pharmacology to safe, effective, and rational drug therapy.

Key Points to Remember

- Pharmacology is the scientific study of drugs and their effects on living organisms.
- Pharmacokinetics describes what the body does to the drug (ADME).
- Pharmacodynamics describes what the drug does to the body.
- Clinical pharmacology applies pharmacological principles to patient care.
- Toxicology focuses on the harmful effects of drugs and chemicals.
- Pharmacovigilance monitors the safety of medicines after they are marketed.
- Pharmacogenomics supports personalized drug therapy based on genetic differences.
- Rational drug use aims to maximize therapeutic benefit while minimizing risks.

Exam Pearls

- Pharmacology = Study of drugs and their interactions with living organisms.
- Pharmacokinetics = ADME (Absorption, Distribution, Metabolism, Excretion).
- Pharmacodynamics = Mechanism of action and drug effects.
- Clinical pharmacology = Safe and rational use of drugs in patients.
- Toxicology = Study of poisons and harmful drug effects.
- Pharmacovigilance = Detection and prevention of adverse drug reactions after marketing.

Branches of Pharmacology

Introduction

Pharmacology is a broad and rapidly evolving biomedical science that encompasses numerous specialized disciplines. Each branch focuses on a particular aspect of drug discovery, development, mechanisms of action, therapeutic applications, safety, or public health. Together, these branches provide the scientific foundation for the rational use of medicines and the advancement of modern healthcare.

Understanding the various branches of pharmacology enables healthcare professionals to appreciate how drugs are discovered, evaluated, prescribed, monitored, and used to improve patient outcomes.

Major Branches of Pharmacology

1. Pharmacokinetics

Definition:

Pharmacokinetics is the study of what the body does to a drug after its administration.

It describes the movement of drugs through the body using the four major processes

known as ADME:

- Absorption
- Distribution
- Metabolism Excretion

Importance

- Determines drug dosage.
- Predicts drug concentration in the body.
- Helps prevent drug accumulation and toxicity.
- Guides dosage adjustments in patients with liver or kidney disease.

2. Pharmacodynamics

Definition:

Pharmacodynamics is the study of what a drug does to the body.

It examines:

- Mechanism of action
- Drug-receptor interactions
- Therapeutic effects
- Adverse effects
- Dose–response relationships

Importance

- Explains how drugs produce their effects.
- Helps select the most effective medication.
- Predicts therapeutic and toxic responses.

3. Clinical Pharmacology

Definition:

Clinical pharmacology applies pharmacological principles to the prevention, diagnosis, and treatment of disease in human patients.

Major Areas

- Rational prescribing
- Drug selection
- Therapeutic drug monitoring
- Individualized drug therapy
- Drug interactions
- Evidence-based medicine

Importance

- Improves patient safety.
- Optimizes therapeutic outcomes.
- Reduces medication errors.

4. Toxicology

Definition:

Toxicology is the study of the harmful effects of drugs, chemicals, and poisons on living organisms.

Areas of Study

- Drug overdose
- Poisoning
- Environmental toxins
- Occupational exposure
- Antidotes
- Prevention of toxicity

Importance

- Identifies toxic substances.
- Guides emergency management.
- Improves patient safety.

5. Chemotherapy

Definition:

Chemotherapy is the use of chemical agents to treat infectious diseases and cancer.

Drug Classes

- Antibiotics
- Antiviral drugs
- Antifungal drugs
- Antiparasitic drugs
- Anticancer agents

Importance

- Eliminates disease-causing microorganisms.
- Treats malignant diseases.
- Improves survival rates.

6. Pharmacotherapeutics

Definition:

Pharmacotherapeutics is the study of the clinical use of drugs for the prevention and treatment of disease.

Focus

- Choosing appropriate medications
- Selecting correct doses
- Monitoring therapeutic response
- Managing adverse effects

Importance

- Promotes rational drug therapy.
- Improves clinical decision-making.

7. Pharmacogenomics

Definition:

Pharmacogenomics studies how genetic variations influence an individual's response to medications.

Applications

- Personalized medicine
- Individualized dosing
- Improved drug efficacy
- Reduced adverse drug reactions

Importance

- Enhances treatment effectiveness.
- Minimizes drug toxicity.

8. Pharmacoepidemiology

Definition:

Pharmacoepi
demiology studies the use and effects of drugs in large populations.

Applications

- Drug utilization studies
- Medication safety monitoring
- Public health research
- Evaluation of prescribing patterns

Importance

- Detects rare adverse effects.
- Supports healthcare policy and drug regulation.

9. Pharmacovigilance

Definition:

Pharmacovigilance is the science of detecting, assessing, understanding, and preventing adverse drug reactions and other medication-related problems.

Activities

- Monitoring drug safety
- Reporting adverse drug reactions
- Evaluating medication risks
- Improving patient safety

Importance

- Ensures continued drug safety after approval.
- Supports regulatory decision-making.

10. Experimental Pharmacology

Definition:

Experimental pharmacology investigates drug actions using laboratory models before clinical use.

Areas

- Animal studies
- Cell culture experiments
- Drug screening
- Mechanism-of-action research

Importance

- Supports drug discovery.
- Evaluates safety and efficacy before human trials.

11. Molecular Pharmacology

Definition:

Molecular pharmacology examines drug actions at the molecular and cellular levels.

Focus

- Cell signaling pathways
- Receptor biology
- Gene regulation
- Molecular targets

Importance

- Facilitates the development of targeted therapies.
- Advances precision medicine.

12. Neuropharmacology

Definition:

Neuropharmacology studies drugs that affect the nervous system.

Examples

- Antidepressants
- Antipsychotics
- Antiepileptic drugs
- Anesthetics
- Opioid analgesics

Importance

Improvesthemanagementofneurologicalandpsychiatric disorders.

13. Cardiovascular Pharmacology

Definition:

Cardiovascular pharmacology focuses on drugs used to diagnose, prevent, and treat diseases of the heart and blood vessels.

Examples

- Antihypertensive drugs
- Antiarrhythmics
- Diuretics
- Antianginal drugs
- Heart failure medications

14. Endocrine Pharmacology

Definition:

Endocrine pharmacology studies medications that influence hormonal function.

Examples

- Insulin
- Oral antidiabetic drugs
- Thyroid medications
- Corticosteroids
- Sex hormones

15. Immunopharmacology

Definition:

Immunopharmacology examines drugs that modify the immune system.

Examples

- Vaccines
- Immunosuppressants
- Monoclonal antibodies
- Immunostimulants

Importance

- Treats autoimmune diseases.
- Prevents organ transplant rejection.
- Supports cancer immunotherapy.

Summary Table

Branch	Main Focus
Pharmacokinetics	What the body does to the drug (ADME)
Pharmacodynamics	What the drug does to the body
Clinical Pharmacology	Drug use in patients
Toxicology	Harmful effects of drugs and poisons
Chemotherapy	Drugs for infections and cancer
Pharmacotherapeutics	Rational treatment with medications
Pharmacogenomics	Genetic influences on drug response
Pharmacoepidemiology	Drug effects in populations
Pharmacovigilance	Monitoring drug safety after marketing
Experimental Pharmacology	Laboratory investigation of drugs
Molecular Pharmacology	Drug action at the molecular level
Neuropharmacology	Drugs affecting the nervous system
Cardiovascular Pharmacology	Drugs affecting the heart and blood vessels
Endocrine Pharmacology	Hormone-related medications
Immunopharmacology	Drugs that modify immune responses

Learning Objectives

- After studying this chapter, you should be able to:
- Define the major branches of pharmacology.
- Differentiate between pharmacokinetics and pharmacodynamics.
- Explain the role of clinical pharmacology in patient care.
- Describe the importance of toxicology and pharmacovigilance.
- Recognize the applications of pharmacogenomics and pharmacoepidemiology.
- Identify specialized fields of pharmacology relevant to modern clinical practice.

Key Points to Remember

- Pharmacology consists of multiple specialized disciplines that together support safe and effective medication use.
- Pharmacokinetics focuses on drug absorption, distribution, metabolism, and excretion (ADME).
- Pharmacodynamics explains drug mechanisms of action and physiological effects.
- Clinical pharmacology applies pharmacological knowledge to optimize patient care.
- Pharmacovigilance is essential for detecting and preventing adverse drug reactions after medicines reach the market.
- Pharmacogenomics enables personalized therapy based on genetic variation.
- Specialized branches such as neuropharmacology, cardiovascular pharmacology, endocrine pharmacology, and immunopharmacology address drug therapy within specific organ systems.

Exam Pearls

- Pharmacokinetics = What the body does to the drug (ADME).
- Pharmacodynamics = What the drug does to the body.
- Clinical Pharmacology = Rational use of drugs in patients.
- Toxicology = Study of harmful effects of drugs and chemicals.
- Pharmacovigilance = Post-marketing monitoring of drug safety.
- Pharmacogenomics = Personalized medicine based on genetic differences.
- Pharmacoepidemiology = Study of drug use and effects in populations.

Drug Nomenclature

Introduction

Drug nomenclature is the standardized system used to identify and classify medications. A single drug may have several different names, each serving a specific purpose during drug development, regulatory approval, prescribing, dispensing, and marketing.

Understanding the different types of drug names is essential for healthcare professionals to ensure accurate prescribing, safe medication administration, effective communication, and prevention of medication errors.

Types of Drug Names

A drug typically has four recognized names:

- Chemical Name
- Generic (Nonproprietary) Name
- Brand (Trade or Proprietary) Name
- Official Name

1. Chemical Name

Definition

The chemical name describes the exact molecular structure and chemical composition of a drug according to the rules established by the International Union of Pure and Applied Chemistry (IUPAC).

Chemical names are often long and complex and are primarily used in research and scientific publications rather than in clinical practice.

Example

Acetaminophen (Paracetamol)

Chemical name:

N-(4-hydroxyphenyl)acetamide

Characteristics

- Describes the chemical structure.
- Assigned before clinical use.
- Used mainly by chemists and researchers.
- Usually difficult to remember.

2. Generic Name (Nonproprietary Name)

Definition

The generic name is the universally accepted, official nonproprietary name assigned to a drug after it has been approved for clinical use.

Generic names are approved by recognized organizations such as the United States Adopted Names (USAN) Council and the International Nonproprietary Names (INN) Programme coordinated by the World Health Organization (WHO).

Healthcare professionals should prescribe medications by their generic names whenever possible because they are universally recognized and reduce confusion.

Examples

Generic Name	Drug Class
Aspirin	NSAID
Amoxicillin	Penicillin antibiotic
Metformin	Antidiabetic
Atenolol	Beta blocker
Furosemide	Loop diuretic
Omeprazole	Proton pump inhibitor
Atorvastatin	Statin

Characteristics

- One generic name for each drug.
- Accepted internationally.
- Less expensive than brand-name products.
- Preferred for prescribing in most healthcare systems.
- Remains the same regardless of the manufacturer.

3. Brand (Trade or Proprietary) Name

Definition

A brand name (trade name) is the commercial name chosen by a pharmaceutical company to market its product.

A single generic drug may be marketed under multiple brand names by different manufacturers

.Examples

Generic Name	Common Brand Name(s)
Acetaminophen	Tylenol®
Ibuprofen	Advil®, Motrin®
Omeprazole	Prilosec®
Atorvastatin	Lipitor®
Metformin	Glucophage®

Characteristics

- Protected by trademark laws.
- Easy to pronounce and remember.
- Different companies may use different brand names.
- Usually more expensive than generic products.

4. Official Name

Definition

The official name is the name listed in an official pharmacopoeia or national formulary, such as the:

- United States Pharmacopeia (USP)
- British Pharmacopoeia (BP)
- European Pharmacopoeia (Ph. Eur.)
- Japanese Pharmacopoeia (JP)

In many cases, the official name is identical to the generic name.

Drug Name Sequence

During drug development, a medication usually receives its names in the following order:

- Chemical name
- Code number (during research)
- Generic (nonproprietary) name
- Brand (trade) name after marketing approval

Generic vs Brand Name

Feature	Generic Name	Brand Name
Ownership	Public	Trademarked by manufacturer
Number of Names	One	May be many
Cost	Usually lower	Usually higher
Standard Worldwide	Yes	No
Prescribing Preference	Preferred	Used for marketing

.Drug Name Stems

Many generic drugnames share common suffixes (stems) that identify their pharmacological class.

Stem	Drug Class	Examples
-pril	ACE inhibitors	Enalapril, Lisinopril
-sartan	Angiotensin II receptor blockers (ARBs)	Losartan, Valsartan
-olol	Beta blockers	Atenolol, Metoprolol
-dipine	Calcium channel blockers	Amlodipine, Nifedipine
-statin	HMG-CoA reductase inhibitors	Atorvastatin, Rosuvastatin
-prazole	Proton pump inhibitors	Omeprazole, Pantoprazole
-cillin	Penicillins	Amoxicillin, Ampicillin
-cycline	Tetracyclines	Doxycycline, Minocycline
-floxacin	Fluoroquinolones	Ciprofloxacin, Levofloxacin
-azole	Azole antifungals	Fluconazole, Ketoconazole
-mab	Monoclonal antibodies	Trastuzumab, Adalimumab

Recognizing these stems helps healthcare professionals quickly identify a drug's class and anticipate its therapeutic effects and adverse reactions.

Importance of Drug Nomenclature

Understanding drug nomenclature helps healthcare professionals to:

- Prescribe medications accurately.
- Prevent medication errors.
- Communicate effectively among healthcare teams.
- Identify drugs within the same pharmacological class.
- Select cost-effective generic alternatives.
- Interpret medicalliterature and treatment guidelines correctly.

Learning Objectives

After studying this chapter, you should be able to:

- Define drug nomenclature.
- Differentiate between chemical, generic, brand, and official names.
- Explain the advantages of prescribing by generic name.
- Recognize common generic drug name stems.
- Identify medications according to their pharmacological class.

Key Points to Remember

- A drug may have chemical, generic, brand, and official names.
- The chemical name describes the molecular structure.
- The generic name is the internationally recognized nonproprietary name and is preferred for prescribing.
- The brand name is a trademark chosen by the manufacturer and may vary between companies.
- The official name appears in recognized pharmacopoeias and is often the same as the generic name.
- Commonsuffixes in generic names often indicate a drug's pharmacological class.

Exam Pearls

- Chemical name: Describes the molecular structure of the drug.
- Generic (nonproprietary) name: Standard international name used in prescribing.
- Brand (trade) name: Commercial name selected by the manufacturer.
- Official name: Name listed in an official pharmacopoeia.
- Generic drugs contain the same active ingredient, strength, dosage form, and therapeutic effect as their brand-name counterparts, although inactive ingredients may differ.
- Learning drug name stems is a high-yield strategy for recognizing drug classes and answering pharmacology examination questions.

Drug Classification

Introduction

Drug classification is the systematic grouping of medications according to shared characteristics such as their source, chemical structure, mechanism of action, therapeutic use, pharmacological effects, or legal status. A single drug may belong to more than one classification system depending on the context.

Understanding drug classification enables healthcare professionals to recognize similarities among medications, predict therapeutic effects and adverse reactions, identify potential drug interactions, and make informed decisions in clinical practice.

Objectives of Drug Classification

Drug classification helps to:

- Organize medications into logical groups.
- Simplify the study of pharmacology.
- Predict drug actions and adverse effects.
- Facilitate rational drug selection.
- Improve communication among healthcare professionals.
- Support safe prescribing and medication management.

Major Methods of Drug Classification

Drugs may be classified according to:

- Source (Origin)
- Chemical Structure
- Mechanism of Action
- Pharmacological Effect
- Therapeutic Use
- Anatomical System (Organ System)
- LegalorRegulatory Status

1. Classification According to Source (Origin)

This classification groups drugs based on where they are obtained.

A. Plant Sources

Drugs derived from plants.

Examples

Drug	**Source**
Morphine	Opium poppy (Papaver somniferum)
Digoxin	Foxglove (Digitalis lanata)
Atropine	Deadly nightshade (Atropa belladonna)
Quinine	Cinchona bark

B. Animal Sources

Drugs obtained from animal tissues or secretions.

Examples

- Insulin (historically from porcine or bovine pancreas)
- Heparin (porcine intestinal mucosa)
- Thyroid hormone (historically from animal thyroid glands)

Note: Many of these products are now manufactured using recombinant DNA technology.

C. Microbial Sources

Produced by microorganisms.

Examples

- Penicillin (Penicillium species)
- Streptomycin (Streptomyces griseus)
- Erythromycin (Saccharopolyspora erythraea)

D. Mineral Sources

Derived from naturally occurring minerals.

Examples

- Magnesium sulfate
- Lithium carbonate
- Ferrous sulfate
- Potassium chloride

E. Synthetic Drugs

Produced entirely by chemical synthesis.

Examples

- Paracetamol (Acetaminophen)
- Metformin
- Omeprazole
- Lidocaine

F. Biotechnology-Derived Drugs

Produced using genetic engineering and biotechnology.

Examples

- Human insulin
- Epoetin alfa
- Monoclonal antibodies Recombinant clotting factors

2. Classification According to Chemical Structure

Drugs with similar chemical structures often have comparable pharmacological properties.

Examples

Chemical Class	Examples
Penicillins	Amoxicillin, Ampicillin
Cephalosporins	Ceftriaxone, Cephalexin
Benzodiazepines	Diazepam, Lorazepam
Corticosteroids	Prednisone, Dexamethasone
Sulfonamides	Sulfamethoxazole

3. Classification According to Mechanism of Action

This system groups drugs by how they produce their effects.

Examples

Mechanism	Drug Examples
ACE inhibitors	Lisinopril, Enalapril
Beta-adrenergic blockers	Atenolol, Metoprolol
Proton pump inhibitors	Omeprazole, Pantoprazole
Calcium channel blockers	Amlodipine, Verapamil
HMG-CoA reductase inhibitors	Atorvastatin, Rosuvastatin

Understanding mechanisms of action helps predict therapeutic effects, contraindications, and potential drug interactions.

4. Classification According to Pharmacological Effect

This method groups drugs according to their physiological effects on the body.

Examples

PharmacologicalEffect	Drug Examples
Analgesics	Morphine, Ibuprofen
Antipyretics	Paracetamol
Anti-inflammatory drugs	Naproxen, Diclofenac
Sedatives	Diazepam
Bronchodilators	Salbutamol

5. Classification According to Therapeutic Use

Drugs are grouped according to the diseases or conditions they treat.

Examples

Therapeutic Class	Examples
Antihypertensive drugs	Lisinopril, Amlodipine
Antidiabetic drugs	Metformin, Insulin
Antibiotics	Amoxicillin, Azithromycin
Antifungal drugs	Fluconazole
Antidepressants	Sertraline
Antiepileptic drugs	Valproate

A single drug may have more than one therapeutic indication.

6. Classification According to Anatomical (Organ) System

The Anatomical Therapeutic Chemical (ATC) Classification System, developed by the World Health Organization (WHO), classifies drugs according to the organ or system on which they primarily act, together with their therapeutic, pharmacological, and chemical characteristics.

Major anatomical groups include:

- Cardiovascular system
- Respiratory system
- Gastrointestinal system
- Central nervous system
- Endocrine system
- Musculoskeletal system
- Genitourinary system
- Anti-infective agents
- Dermatological drugs
- Ophthalmic preparations

This system is widely used in clinical practice, research, and pharmacovigilance.

7. Classification According to Legal or Regulatory Status

Drugs may also be classified according to how they are regulated.

Prescription-Only Medicines (POM)

Require authorization from a licensed healthcare professional.

Examples

- Insulin
- Warfarin
- Amoxicillin

Over-the-Counter (OTC) Medicines

Can be purchased without a prescription when used according to labeled directions.

Examples

- Paracetamol (Acetaminophen)
- Ibuprofen (at approved OTC doses)
- Antacids

Controlled Substances

Medications with potential for abuse or dependence that are subject to additional legal controls.

Examples

- Morphine
- Fentanyl
- Methylphenidate

Regulations vary by country.

Why Drugs May Belong to Multiple Classes

Many medications fit into more than one classification.

Example: Aspirin

- Source: Synthetic
- Chemical class: Salicylate
- Mechanism: Cyclooxygenase (COX) inhibitor
- Pharmacological effect: Analgesic, antipyretic, anti-inflammatory, antiplatelet
- Therapeutic use: Pain relief, fever reduction, prevention of thrombotic cardiovascular events

Recognizing multiple classifications helps healthcare professionals understand the full range of a drug's clinical applications.

Learning Objectives

After studying this chapter, you should be able to:

- Define drug classification.
- Describe the major methods of classifying drugs.
- Differentiate between pharmacological, therapeutic, and mechanistic classifications.
- Explain why a single drug may belong to more than one classification.
- Applydrug classification principles to clinical decision-making.

Key Points to Remember

- Drug classification organizes medications into meaningful groups based on shared characteristics.
- Drugs can be classified by source, chemical structure, mechanism of action, pharmacological effect, therapeutic use, anatomical system, or legal status.
- A medication often belongs to several classifications simultaneously.
- Mechanism-based classification is particularly useful for predicting efficacy, adverse effects, and drug interactions.
- The WHO Anatomical Therapeutic Chemical (ATC) Classification System is an internationally recognized system for categorizing medications.

Exam Pearls

- Source classification: Plant, animal, microbial, mineral, synthetic, or biotechnology-derived.
- Mechanism of action: Explains how a drug works (e.g., ACE inhibitor, beta blocker).
- Therapeutic classification: Explains what condition a drug treats (e.g., antihypertensive, antidiabetic).
- Pharmacological classification: Describes the drug's physiological effect (e.g., analgesic, bronchodilator).
- A single drug may belong to multiple classifications, making it important to understand each perspective for safe and effective patient care.

Sources of Drugs

Introduction

Drugs are obtained from a wide variety of natural and synthetic sources. Throughout history, medicinal substances were primarily derived from plants, animals, and minerals. Advances in chemistry, microbiology, molecular biology, and biotechnology have greatly expanded the range of available medications, leading to the development of safer, more effective, and more targeted therapies.

Understanding the sources of drugs helps healthcare professionals appreciate their origin, production methods, pharmacological properties, and clinical applications.

Definition

A source of drugs refers to the origin from which a drug or its active ingredient is obtained. Drugs may be derived from natural sources, synthesized chemically, or produced through biotechnology.

Classification of Drug Sources

Drugs are broadly classified according to their origin into:

1. Plant Sources
2. Animal Sources
3. Microbial Sources
4. Mineral Sources
5. Marine Sources
6. Synthetic Sources
7. Semisynthetic Sources
8. Biotechnology (Recombinant DNA) Sources

1. Plant Sources

Plants have been used for medicinal purposes for thousands of years and continue to provide many important therapeutic agents.

Advantages

- Rich source of biologically active compounds
- Historically important in drug discovery
- Many modern drugs originated from medicinal plants

Examples

Drug	Plant Source	Clinical Use
Morphine	Papaver somniferum(Opiumpoppy)	Severe pain
Codeine	Opium poppy	Cough suppressio
Digoxin	Digitalis lanata (Foxglove)	Heart failure.
Atropine	Atropa belladonna	Bradycardia.
Quinine	Cinchona bark	Malaria
Pilocarpine	Pilocarpus species	Glaucoma, xerostomia
Vincristine	Madagascar	Cancer chemotherapy
Paclitaxel	periwinkle	Cancer chemotherapy

2. Animal Sources

Some drugs are obtained from animal tissues, organs, or body fluids. Although many have been replaced by recombinant products, several remain in clinical use.

Examples

Drug	Animal Source	Clinical Use
Heparin	Porcine intestinal mucosa	Anticoagulation
Protamine	Salmon sperm	Heparin reversal
Pancreatic enzyme	Porcine pancreas	Pancreatic enzyme
Antivenoms	Horse or sheep serum	Treatment of venomous bit

Note: Insulin was historically obtained from bovine and porcine pancreas but is now produced predominantly by recombinant DNA technology.

3. Microbial Sources

Many important medications are produced by bacteria and fungi, especially antibiotics.

Examples

Drug	Microorganism	Clinical Use
Penicillin	Penicillium species	Bacterial infections
Streptomycin	Streptomyces griseus	Tuberculosis, other infections
Erythromycin	Saccharopolyspora erythraea	Respiratory and skin infection
Vancomycin	Amycolatopsis oriental	Serious Gram-positive infections
Cyclosporine	Tolypocladium inflatum	Immunosuppression

4. Mineral Sources

Minerals provide essential therapeutic agents used in various medical conditions.

Examples

Drug	Source	Clinical Use
Magnesium sulfate	Mineral deposits	Eclampsia, magnesium deficiency
Ferrous sulfate	Iron	Iron-deficiency anemia
Potassium chloride	Potassium salts	Hypokalemia
Lithium carbonate	Lithium minerals	Bipolar disorder
Calcium carbonate	Limestone	Calcium supplementation, antacid

5. Marine Sources

Marine organisms are a valuable source of unique bioactive compounds used in modern medicine.

Examples

Drug	Marine Source	Clinical Use
Cytarabine	Marine sponge derivatives	Leukemia
Ziconotide	Cone snail (Conus magus) venom	Severe chronic pain
Trabectedin	Sea squirt (Ecteinascidia turbinata)	Soft tissue sarcoma, ovarian cancer

Marinenatural productscontinuetobeinvestigatedforantimicrobial,anticancer,andanti-inflammatory activities.

6. Synthetic Sources

Synthetic drugs are manufactured entirely by chemical synthesis in laboratories or pharmaceutical industries.

Advantages

- High purity
- Large-scale production
- Consistent quality
- Lower production costs for many drugs
- Reduced dependence on natural resources

Examples

Drug	**Clinical Use**
Paracetamol (Acetaminophen)	Pain and fever
Lidocaine	Local anesthesia
Omeprazole	Peptic ulcer disease, GERD
Metformin	Type 2 diabetes mellitus
Amlodipine	Hypertension

7. Semisynthetic Sources

Semisynthetic drugs are produced by chemically modifying naturally occurring compounds to improve their pharmacological properties.

Advantages

- Increased effectiveness
- Improved stability
- Better absorption
- Reduced toxicity
- Expanded antimicrobial spectrum

Examples

Parent NaturalCompound	Semisynthetic Drug
Penicillin G	Amoxicillin
Penicillin G	Ampicillin
Erythromycin	Clarithromycin
Morphine	Hydromorphone
Tetracycline	Doxycycline

8. Biotechnology (Recombinant DNA) Sources

Modern biotechnology uses genetically engineered microorganisms or mammalian cell lines to produce highly purified therapeutic proteins and biologic agents.

Advantages

- High purity
- Reduced risk of contamination
- Consistent quality
- Large-scale production
- Improved safety and efficacy

Examples

Drug	Clinical Use
Recombinant human insulin	Diabetes mellitus
Epoetin alfa	Anemia associated with chronic kidney disease
Filgrastim	Neutropenia
Recombinant factor VIII	Hemophilia A
Alteplase (tPA)	Acute ischemic stroke, mycardial infarction
Monoclonal antibodies (e.g., trastuzumab,adalimumab)	Cancer and autoimmune diseases

Emerging Sources of Drugs

Advances in biomedical research continue to identify new sources of therapeutic agents, including:

- Gene therapy
- Cell therapy
- RNA-based therapeutics (e.g., small interfering RNA and messenger RNA)
- CRISPR-based therapies
- Nanomedicine
- Artificial intelligence-assisted drug discovery

These innovations are shaping the future of personalized medicine and targeted treatment.

Summary Table

Source	**Examples**
Plant	Morphine, Digoxin, Atropine, Quinine
Animal	Heparin, Protamine, Pancreatic enzymes
Mic	Penicillin, Streptomycin, Vancomycin
Mineral	Magnesium sulfate, Ferrous sulfate, Lithium carbonate
Marine	Cytarabine, Ziconotide, Trabectedin
Synthetic	Paracetamol, Metformin, Omeprazole
Semisynthetic	Amoxicillin, Doxycycline, Clarithromycin
Biotechnology	Recombinant insulin, Epoetin alfa, Monoclonal antibodies

Emerging Sources of Drugs

Advances in biomedical research continue to identify new sources of therapeutic agents, including:

- Gene therapy
- Cell therapy
- RNA-based therapeutics (e.g., small interfering RNA and messenger RNA)
- CRISPR-based therapies
- Nanomedicine
- Artificial intelligence-assisted drug discovery

These innovations are shaping the future of personalized medicine and targeted treatment.

Exam Pearls

- Morphine → Opium poppy (Papaver somniferum)
- Digoxin → Foxglove (Digitalis lanata)
- Atropine → Deadly nightshade (Atropa belladonna)
- Quinine → Cinchona bark
- Penicillin → Penicillium species
- Heparin → Porcine intestinal mucosa
- Recombinant human insulin → Produced by recombinant DNA technology
- Amoxicillin → Semisynthetic penicillin
- Ziconotide → Cone snail venom
- Monoclonal antibodies → Produced using biotechnology and genetic engineering

Routes of Drug Administration

Introduction

The route of drug administration refers to the pathway by which a drug is delivered into the body to produce its therapeutic effect. The choice of route depends on several factors, including the drug's physicochemical properties, the desired onset and duration of action, the patient's clinical condition, convenience, safety, and the intended site of action.

Selecting the appropriate route of administration is essential for maximizing therapeutic efficacy while minimizing adverse effects and ensuring patient compliance.

Definition

A route of drug administration is the method by which a drug is introduced into the body to achieve a desired therapeutic effect.

Factors Influencing the Choice of Route

The choice of route depends on:

- Patient's age and clinical condition
- Emergency versus non-emergency situations
- Desired onset and duration of action
- Drug stability
- Drug absorption characteristics
- First-pass hepatic metabolism
- Patient compliance
- Local versus systemic effects
- Cost and convenience

I. Enteral Routes

Enteral administration delivers drugs through the gastrointestinal tract.

A. Oral Route (PO)

Definition

The drug is swallowed and absorbed primarily from the stomach or small intestine.

Advantages

- Most convenient
- Safe
- Economical
- Suitable for long-term therapy
- Self-administration possible

Disadvantages

- Slow onset of action
- Subject to first-pass metabolism
- Not suitable for unconscious or vomiting patients
- Drug degradation by gastric acid or digestive enzymes

Examples

- Paracetamol
- Amoxicillin
- Metformin
- Aspirin

B. Sublingual Route

Definition

The drug is placed beneath the tongue and absorbed through the oral mucosa directly into the systemic circulation.

Advantages

- Rapid onset
- Avoids first-pass metabolism
- Useful during emergencies
- Easy administration

Disadvantages

- Only small doses can be administered
- Some drugs have unpleasant taste
- Patient must not swallow immediately

Examples

- Nitroglycerin
- Isosorbide dinitrate

C. Buccal Route

Definition

The drug is placed between the cheek and gum for absorption through the buccal mucosa.

Advantages

- Avoids first-pass metabolism
- Sustained absorption
- Convenient

Examples

- Nicotine gum
- Buccal fentanyl

D. Rectal Route

Definition

Drugs are administered into the rectum as suppositories, enemas, or creams.

Advantages

- Useful in unconscious or vomiting patients
- Partial avoidance of first-pass metabolism
- Local or systemic effects

Disadvantages

- Variable absorption
- Patient discomfort
- Less acceptable to some patients

Examples

- Diazepam suppository
- Glycerin suppository
- Acetaminophen suppository

II. Parenteral Routes

Parenteral administration bypasses the gastrointestinal tract and usually involves injection.

A. Intravenous (IV)

Definition

Drug is injected directly into a vein.

Advantages

- Immediate onset
- 100% bioavailability
- Precise control of dosage
- Suitable for emergencies

Disadvantages

- Requires trained personnel
- Risk of infection
- Irreversible once administered
- Higher cost

Examples

- Ceftriaxone
- Heparin
- Vancomycin
- Alteplase

B. Intramuscular (IM)

Definition

Drug is injected into skeletal muscle.

Advantages

- Faster absorption than subcutaneous injections
- Suitable for depot preparations
- Moderate drug volumes can be administered

Disadvantages

- Painful
- Risk of nerve injury
- Bleeding risk in anticoagulated patients

Examples

- Vaccines
- Ceftriaxone
- Vitamin B12
- Benzathine penicillin

C. Subcutaneous (SC)

Definition

Drug is injected into the subcutaneous tissue.

Advantages

- Slow, sustained absorption
- Self-administration possible
- Suitable for biologic drugs

Disadvantages

- Small injection volume
- Slower onset than IV
- Local irritation possible

Examples

- Insulin
- Low-molecular-weight heparin
- GLP-1 receptor agonists

D. Intradermal (ID)

Definition

Drug is injected into the dermis.

Uses

- Allergy testing
- Tuberculin skin test (Mantoux test)
- Selected vaccines

Advantages

- Localized effect
- Small drug dose required

E. Other Specialized Parenteral Routes

These routes are used for specific clinical indications.

Route	Common Uses
Intrathecal	Spinal anesthesia, chemotherapy
Epidural	Labor analgesia, postoperative pain control
Intra-articular	Corticosteroid injection into joints
Intraosseous	Emergency vascular access
Intraperitoneal	Dialysis, chemotherapy

III. Topical Routes

Topical administration delivers drugs directly to the skin or mucous membranes.

A. Cutaneous Route

Examples

- Hydrocortisone cream
- Mupirocin ointment
- Antifungal creams

Advantages

- Local effect
- Minimal systemic adverse effects

B. Transdermal Route

Drug is delivered across intact skin using adhesive patches.

Advantages

- Sustained drug release
- Avoids first-pass metabolism
- Improves patient compliance

Examples

- Nitroglycerin patch
- Nicotine patch
- Fentanyl patch
- Scopolamine patch

C. Ophthalmic Route

Examples:

- Timolol eye drops
- Artificial tears
- Ciprofloxacin eye drops

D. Otic Route

Examples:

- Ciprofloxacin ear drops
- Carbamide peroxide

E. Nasal Route

Examples:

- Oxymetazoline
- Fluticasone nasal spray
- Desmopressin

Advantages include rapid absorption and avoidance of first-pass metabolism.

F. Vaginal Route

Examples:

- Clotrimazole pessaries
- Estrogen cream

Used for local or systemic therapy.

IV. Inhalational Route

Drugs are inhaled into the respiratory tract.

Advantages

- Rapid onset
- Direct delivery to lungs
- Smaller doses required
- Reduced systemic adverse effects

Disadvantages

Requires proper inhaler technique
Variable drug deposition

Examples

- Salbutamol
- Budesonide
- Ipratropium
- Sevoflurane

Learning Objectives

After studying this chapte, you should be able to:

- Define the routes of drug administration.
- Classify drugs according to their route of administration.
- Compare the advantages and disadvantages of each route.
- Identify factors influencing route selection.
- Selectthe most appropriate route for different clinical situations.

Key Points to Remember

- The routeofadministrationinfluences drug absorption, onset of action,
- bioavailability, and therapeutic outcome.
- Oral administration is the most common and convenient route but is subject to first-pass metabolism.
- Intravenous administration provides immediate drug delivery with 100% bioavailability.
- Sublingual and transdermal routes avoid first-pass hepatic metabolism. Inhalational therapy delivers drugs rapidly to the lungs and is particularly useful for respiratory diseases.
- The choice of route depends on the patient's condition, drug characteristics, desired therapeutic effect, and clinical urgency.

Exam Pearls

- Intravenous (IV): Fastest onset and 100% bioavailability.
- Oral route: Most convenient but subject to first-pass hepatic metabolism.
- Sublingual route: Rapid absorption and bypasses first-pass metabolism (e.g., nitroglycerin).
- Rectal route: Useful in unconscious or vomiting patients and partially avoids first-pass metabolism.
- Subcutaneous route: Commonly used for insulin and low-molecular-weight heparin.
- Intradermal route: Used for allergy testing and the Mantoux (tuberculin) test.
- Transdermal patches: Provide sustained drug release while avoiding first-pass metabolism.
- Inhalation route: Preferred for asthma because it delivers medication directly to the lungs with rapid onset and fewer systemic adverse effects.

Drug Receptors

Introduction

Drug receptors are specialized macromolecules, usually proteins, that interact with drugs to produce biological responses. Most drugs exert their therapeutic and adverse effects by binding to specific receptors located on the cell surface, within the cytoplasm, or inside the nucleus. The interaction between a drug and its receptor initiates a series of biochemical and physiological events that ultimately result in the desired pharmacological effect.

Understanding drug receptors is fundamental to pharmacology because it explains how drugs work, why they differ in potency and efficacy, how adverse effects occur, and how rational drug therapy is designed.

Definition

A drug receptor is a specific cellular protein or macromolecule that selectively binds a drug or endogenous ligand and initiates a biological response.

The natural substances that normally bind to receptors are called endogenous ligands, such as neurotransmitters, hormones, and autacoids.

Examples include:

- Acetylcholine → Muscarinic and nicotinic receptors
- Epinephrine (adrenaline) → Alpha and beta adrenergic receptors
- Insulin → Insulin receptor
- Cortisol → Glucocorticoid receptor

Characteristics of Drug Receptors

Drug receptors possess several important properties:

- **Specificity**: Each receptor preferentially binds certain drugs or endogenous ligands.
- **Affinity**: The strength with which a drug binds to its receptor.
- **Selectivity**: Drugs often interact more strongly with one receptor subtype than with others.
- **Saturability**: A finite number of receptors are available; once occupied, increasing the drug dose does not increase receptor binding.
- **Reversibility**: Most drug-receptor interactions are reversible, although some drugs bind irreversibly.

Functions of Drug Receptors

Drugreceptors areresponsiblefor:

- Recognizing signaling molecules.
- Initiating intracellular signaling pathways.
- Regulating physiological functions. Producing therapeutic effects.
- Mediating adverse drug reactions. Maintaining normal cellular communication.

Types of Drug Receptors

Drug receptors are classified into four major families.

1. Ligand-Gated Ion Channels (Ionotropic Receptors) Definition

These receptors are membrane proteins that open or close ion channels when activated by a ligand.

Characteristics

- Very rapid response (milliseconds)
- Control movement of ions across cell membranes
- Important in neurotransmission

Examples

Receptor	Endogenous Ligand	Major Function
Nicotinic acetylcholine receptor	Acetylcholine	Skeletal muscle contraction
GABA_A receptor	GABA	Inhibitory neurotransmission
NMDA receptor	Glutamate	Learning and memory
Glycine receptor	Glycine	Spinal cord inhibition

Clinical Examples

- Benzodiazepines enhance GABA receptor activity.
- Neuromuscular blocking agents act on nicotinic receptors.

2. G Protein-Coupled Receptors (GPCRs)

Definition

GPCRs are membrane receptors that activate intracellular G proteins following ligand binding.

Characteristics

- Most common receptor family
- Response within seconds to minutes
- Regulate numerous physiological functions

Examples

Receptor	Major Function
β_1-Adrenergic receptor	Increases heart rate and contractility
β_2-Adrenergic receptor	Bronchodilation
α_1-Adrenergic receptor	Vasoconstriction
Muscarinic receptors	Parasympathetic responses
Histamine H_1 receptor	Allergic reactions

Clinical Examples

- Salbutamol stimulates β_2 receptors.
- Propranolol blocks β receptors.
- Atropine blocks muscarinic receptors.

3. Enzyme-Linked Receptors

Definition

These receptors possess intrinsic enzyme activity or are directly associated with enzymes.

Characteristics

- Usually protein kinases
- Activated by hormones and growth factors
- Response occurs within minutes to hours

Examples

Receptor	Ligand
Insulin receptor	Insulin
Epidermal growthfactorreceptor(EGFR)	EGF
Platelet-derived growthfactorreceptor	PDGF

Clinical Examples

- Insulin lowers blood glucose by activating its receptor.
- Targeted anticancer drugs inhibit abnormal receptor tyrosine kinases.

4. Intracellular (Nuclear) Receptors

Definition

These receptors are located within the cytoplasm or nucleus and regulate gene transcription after binding lipid-soluble drugs or hormones.

Characteristics

- Slow onset (hours to days)
- Long-lasting effects
- Influence protein synthesis

Examples

Receptor	Ligand
Glucocorticoid receptor	Cortisol, Prednisone
Thyroid hormonereceptor	Thyroxine (T_4)
Estrogen receptor	Estrogen
Vitamin D receptor	Calcitriol

Clinical Examples

- Corticosteroids reduce inflammation by altering gene expression.
- Thyroid hormones regulate metabolism through nuclear receptors.

Drug–Receptor Interaction

Drug action depends on the interaction between the drug and its receptor.

The interaction may result in:

- Activation of the receptor (agonism)
- Partial activation (partial agonism)
- Blockade of the receptor (antagonism)
- Reduction of constitutive receptor activity (inverse agonism)

The magnitude of the response depends on:

- Drug concentration
- Affinity
- Intrinsic efficacy
- Number of available receptors

Receptor Regulation

Cells regulate receptor numbers in response to prolonged stimulation or blockade.

Upregulation

An increase in receptor number.

Occurs after prolonged receptor blockade.

Example

Long-term beta-blocker therapy increases β -adrenergic receptor density.

Downregulation

A decrease in receptor number due to prolonged stimulation.

Example

Continuous exposure to

β_2 agonists may reduce receptor responsiveness.

Spare Receptors

Some tissues possess more receptors than are necessary to produce a maximal response.

These spare receptors allow maximal effects even when only a fraction of receptors are occupied.

Clinical significance:

- Increased sensitivity to agonists.
- Maximal response achieved before all receptors are occupied.

Desensitization and Tachyphylaxis

Desensitization

Gradual reduction in receptor responsiveness during continuous drug exposure.

Tachyphylaxis

Rapid development of decreased responsiveness after repeated administration over a short period.

Examples:

- Topical nasal decongestants (e.g., oxymetazoline)
- Indirect sympathomimetics

Clinical Importance of Drug Receptors

Understanding receptors helps healthcare professionals to:

- Select appropriate medications.
- Predict therapeutic responses.
- Understand adverse drug reactions.
- Anticipate drug interactions.
- Develop targeted therapies.
- Individualize treatment.

Learning Objectives

After studying this chapter, you should be able to:

- Define drug receptors.
- Describe the characteristics of drug receptors.
- Classify the major receptor families.
- Explain receptor regulation, spare receptors, desensitization, and tachyphylaxis.
- Relate receptor functionto clinical pharmacology and therapeutic drug use.

Key Points to Remember

- Most drugs exert their effectsbyinteracting with specific receptors.
- Drug receptors are usually proteins located on the cell membrane, in the cytoplasm, or within the nucleus.
- The four major receptor families are ligand-gated ion channels, G protein-coupled receptors, enzyme-linked receptors, and intracellular (nuclear) receptors.
- Affinity refers to the strength of drug-receptor binding, whereas efficacy refers to the ability of the drug to produce a biological response after binding.
- Upregulation occurs after prolonged receptor blockade, whereas downregulation follows prolonged receptor stimulation.
- Spare receptors allow maximal responses without complete receptor occupancy.
- Desensitization and tachyphylaxis reduce responsiveness during repeated or continuous drug exposure.

Exam Pearls

- Ligand-gated ion channels: Fastest receptor responses (milliseconds).
- G protein-coupled receptors (GPCRs): Largest receptor family and target of many clinically important drugs.
- Enzyme-linked receptors: Include receptor tyrosine kinases such as the insulin receptor.
- Intracellular receptors: Activated by lipid-soluble hormones and drugs; regulate gene transcription.
- Affinity = Ability of a drug to bind to its receptor.
- Efficacy = Ability of a drug to activate the receptor and produce a maximal effect.
- Upregulation follows prolonged receptor blockade; downregulation follows prolonged receptor stimulation.
- Spare receptors increase tissue sensitivity to agonists.

Mechanisms of Drug Action

Introduction

The mechanism of drug action describes the specific biochemical and physiological processes through which a drug produces its therapeutic effects. Understanding how drugs work is fundamental to pharmacology, as it enables healthcare professionals to predict therapeutic responses, adverse effects, drug interactions, and contraindications.

Most drugs act by interacting with specific molecular targets such as receptors, enzymes, ion channels, transport proteins, or nucleic acids. Some drugs also exert their effects through physical or chemical actions without binding to a receptor.

A thorough understanding of drug mechanisms forms the basis for rational prescribing and evidence-based clinical practice.

Definition

The mechanism of drug action refers to the specific molecular interaction through which a drug produces its pharmacological effect.

Drug action generally involves one or more of the following:

- Binding to receptors
- Modulating enzymes
- Altering ion channels
- Affecting transport proteins
- Interacting with nucleic acids
- Producing physical or chemical effects

Major Mechanisms of Drug Action

Most drugs produce their effects through one of six major mechanisms.

1. Action on Receptors
2. Action on Enzymes
3. Action on Ion Channels
4. Action on Transport Proteins
5. Action on Nucleic Acids 6. Physical and Chemical Actions

1. Action on Receptors

The majority of therapeutic drugs exert their effects by binding to specific receptors located on cell membranes or within cells.

When a drug binds to its receptor, it may:

- Activate the receptor (agonist)
- Partially activate the receptor (partial agonist)
- Block receptor activation (antagonist)
- Reduce constitutive receptor activity (inverse agonist)

Examples

Drug	Target Receptor	Action
Salbutamol	β_2-Adrenergic receptor	Agonist causing bronchodilation
Propranolol	β_1/β_2-Adrenergic receptors	Antagonist reducing heart rate
Atropine	Muscarinic receptor	Competitive antagonist
Morphine	μ-Opioid receptor	Agonist producing analgesia

2. Action on Enzymes

Many drugs act by inhibiting or activating enzymes involved in physiological pathways.

Enzyme inhibition may be:

- Reversible
- Irreversible

Examples

Drug	Enzyme	Result
Aspirin	Cyclooxygenase (COX)	Decreases prostaglandin synthesis
Omeprazole	H^+/K^+-ATPase	Reduces gastric acid secretion
Neostigmine	Acetylcholinesterase	Increases acetylcholine concentration
Allopurinol	Xanthine oxidase	Reduces uric acid production
ACE inhibitors	Angiotensin-converting enzyme	Decrease angiotensin II formation

3. Action on Ion Channels

Certain drugs modify the opening or closing of ion channels, thereby altering cellular excitability.

Ion channels regulate the movement of:

- Sodium (Na^+)
- Potassium (K^+)
- Calcium (Ca^{2+})
- Chloride (Cl^-)

Examples

Drug	Channel	Clinical Effect
Lidocaine	Voltage-gated sodium channels	Local anesthesia
Verapamil	L-type calciumchannels	Decreases cardiac contractility
Amlodipine	L-type calciumchannels	Vasodilation
Amiodarone	Potassium channels	Antiarrhythmic action

4. Action on Transport Proteins

Some drugs inhibit or stimulate transport proteins responsible for moving substances across cell membranes.

Examples

Drug	Transport Protein	Ef fect
Fluoxetine	Serotonin transporter(SERT)	Increases serotonin levels
Digoxin	Na^+/K^+-ATPase	Increases intracellular calcium
SGLT2 inhibitors	Sodium-glucose cotransporter 2	Increase urinary glucose excretion
Furosemide	Na^+-K^+-$2Cl^-$ cotransporter	Promotes diuresis

5. Action on Nucleic Acids

Certain drugs interfere with DNA or RNA synthesis, replication, or transcription.

These drugs are commonly used in oncology and infectious diseases.

Examples

Drug	Target	Clinical Use
Methotrexate	DNA synthesis	Cancer, autoimmune diseases
Doxorubicin	DNA intercalation	Cancer chemotherapy
Ciprofloxacin	Bacterial DNA gyrase	Bacterial infections
Acyclovir	Viral DNA polymerase	Herpes virus infections
Rifampicin	Bacterial RNA polymerase	Tuberculosis

6. Physical and Chemical Actions

Some drugs produce therapeutic effects without interacting with specific receptors.

A. Physical Actions

Examples:

Drug	Mechanism
Activated charcoal	Adsorbs toxins in the gastrointestinal tract
Mannitol	Osmotic diuresis
Bulk-forming laxatives	Increase stool volume

B. Chemical Actions

Examples:

Drug	Mechanism
Antacids	Neutralize gastric acid
Chelating agents (EDTA, Dimercaprol)	Bind heavy metals
Sodium bicarbonate	Neutralizes metabolic acidosis

Selectivity of Drug Action

Most drugs are selective, meaning they preferentially act on one receptor or

molecular target.

However, no drug is completely selective.

As the dose increases:

- Selectivity decreases.
- Adverse effects become more likely.
- Additional receptors or targets may be affected.

Therapeutic Effects vs Adverse Effects

The same mechanism responsible for therapeutic effects may also produce adverse effects.

Example

Beta blockers

Therapeutic effect:

- Reduce heart rate.
- Lower blood pressure.

Adverse effect:

- Bronchoconstriction in susceptible patients.
- Bradycardia.
- Fatigue.

Factors Influencing Drug Action

Drug response may vary depending on:

- Age
- Body weight
- Sex
- Genetic factors
- Liver function
- Kidney function
- Pregnancy
- Drug interactions
- Disease states
- Receptor sensitivity

Clinical Importance

Knowledge of drug mechanisms helps clinicians to:

- Choose the most appropriate medication.
- Predict therapeutic outcomes.
- Anticipate adverse drug reactions.
- Understand drug interactions.
- Manage poisoning and overdose.
- Develop targeted treatment strategies.

Summary Table

Mechanism	Target	Examples
Receptor interaction	Receptors	Salbutamol, Atropine , Morphine
Enzyme inhibition	Enzymes	Aspirin, Omeprazole, Allopurinol
Ion channel modulation	Ion channels	Lidocaine, Verapamil, Amiodarone
Transport protein modulation	Transporters	Fluoxetine, Digoxin, Furosemide
Nucleic acid interaction	DNA /RNA	Methotrexate, Ciprofloxacin, Acyclovir
Physical/Chemical action	Non-receptor mechanisms	Activated charcoal, Antacids, Mannitol

Learning Objectives

After studying this chapter, you should be able to:

- Define the mechanism of drug action.
- Describe the major molecular targets of drugs.
- Differentiate between receptor-mediated and non-receptor-mediated drug actions.
- Explain how drugs modify enzymes, ion channels, transport proteins, and nucleic acids.
- Apply knowledge of drug mechanisms to clinical pharmacology and rational prescribing.

Key Points to Remember

- The mechanism of drug action explains how a drug produces its pharmacological effect .
- Most drugs act on receptors, enzymes, ion channels, transport proteins, or nucleic acids.
- Some drugs act through physical or chemical mechanisms without binding to receptors.
- Drug selectivity improves therapeutic efficacy and reduces adverse effects but is usually dose dependent.
- Understanding drug mechanisms helps predict therapeutic effects, adverse reactions, contraindications, and drug interactions.

Exam Pearls

- Most drugs act by binding to specific receptors.
- Aspirin irreversibly inhibits cyclooxygenase (COX).
- Omeprazole inhibits the H^+/K^+-ATPase proton pump.
- Lidocaine blocks voltage-gated sodium channels.
- Verapamil and amlodipine block L-type calcium channels.
- Fluoxetine inhibits the serotonin transporter (SERT).
- Ciprofloxacin inhibits bacterial DNA gyrase.
- Activated charcoal acts by adsorbing toxins, not by receptor interaction.
- Antacids neutralize gastric acid through a chemical mechanism.
- Selectivity is relative, not absolute—higher doses often increase off-target effects.

Agonists and Antagonists

Introduction

The interaction between drugs and receptors is a fundamental concept in pharmacology. Most drugs exert their effects by binding to specific receptors and either activating them or preventing their activation. Drugs that activate receptors are called agonists, whereas drugs that block receptor activation are known as antagonists.

Understanding the differences between agonists and antagonists is essential for predicting drug responses, selecting appropriate therapies, understanding adverse effects, and interpreting dose-response relationships.

Definitions

Agonist

An agonist is a drug that binds to a receptor and activates it, producing a biological response.

An agonist possesses:

- Affinity – the ability to bind to a receptor.
- Intrinsic efficacy (intrinsic activity) – the ability to activate the receptor and produce a response.

Antagonist

An antagonist is a drug that binds to a receptor without activating it and prevents an agonist or endogenous ligand from producing its effect.

An antagonist possesses:

- Affinity
- No intrinsic efficacy

Drug–Receptor Interaction

The pharmacological response depends on two important properties:

Property	Definition
Affinity	Ability of a drug to bind to a receptor
Efficacy (Intrinsic Activity)	Ability of a drug to activate the receptor after binding

Comparison

Drug Type	Af finity	Ef ficacy
Full agonist	Yes	High
Partial agonist	Yes	Moderate
Antagonist	Yes	None
Inverse agonist	Yes	Negative

Types of Agonists

1. Full Agonist

Definition

A full agonist binds to a receptor and produces the maximum possible biological response, even when not all receptors are occupied.

Characteristics

- High affinity
- High efficacy
- Produces maximal response

Examples

Drug	Receptor
Morphine	μ-Opioid receptor
Epinephrine	Adrenergic receptors
Salbutamol	β_2-Adrenergic receptor
Acetylcholine	Muscarinic and nicotinic receptors

2. Partial Agonist

Definition

A partial agonist binds to the receptor but produces a submaximal response, even when all receptors are occupied.

Characteristics

- High affinity
- Lower efficacy than a full agonist
- Can reduce the effect of a full agonist by competing for the same receptor

Examples

Drug	Receptor
Buprenorphine	μ-Opioid receptor
Aripiprazole	Dopamine D_2 receptor
Pindolol	β-Adrenergic receptor

Clinical Importance

Partial agonists may:

- Produce sufficient therapeutic effects.
- Reduce adverse effects.
- Prevent excessive receptor stimulation.

3. Inverse Agonist

Definition

An inverse agonist binds to the same receptor as an agonist but reduces the receptor's basal (constitutive) activity, producing the opposite effect of an agonist.

Characteristics

- Has affinity
- Produces negative efficacy
- Requires receptors with constitutive activity

Examples

- Some antihistamines acting at H_1 receptors
- Certain beta-blockers
- Some benzodiazepine receptor ligands (primarily of pharmacological interest)

Types of Antagonists

Antagonists are classified according to how they inhibit receptor activation.

1. Competitive (Reversible) Antagonist

Definition

A competitive antagonist binds reversibly to the same receptor site as the agonist .

Increasing the concentration of the agonist can overcome the blockade.

Characteristics

- Reversible binding
- Rightward shift of the dose-response curve
- Maximal response can still be achieved

Examples

Antagonist	**Agonist Blocked**
Atropine	Acetylcholine
Propranolol	Epinephrine, norepinephrine
Naloxone	Opioids
Flumazenil	Benzodiazepines

Clinical Example

Naloxone rapidly reverses opioid overdose by competitively displacing opioids from μ-opioid receptors.

2. Noncompetitive Antagonist

Definition

A noncompetitive antagonist binds irreversibly to the receptor or binds to a different (allosteric) site, reducing receptor activation regardless of agonist concentration.

Characteristics

- Cannot be overcome by increasing agonist concentration
- Decreases maximal response
- Longer duration of action

Examples

Drug	Target
Phenoxybenzamine	α-Adrenergic receptors (irreversible antagonist)
Ketamine*	NMDA receptor (noncompetitive antagonist)

*Ketamine binds within the NMDA receptor ion channel and is commonly classified as a noncompetitive NMDA receptor antagonist.

3. Physiological (Functional) Antagonism

Definition

Two drugs act on different receptors to produce opposite physiological effects.

Example

Drug	Ef fect
Epinephrine	Bronchodilation
Histamine	Bronchoconstriction

Although they act on different receptors, the physiological effects oppose each other.

4. Chemical Antagonism

Definition

One substance chemically combines with another drug, reducing or abolishing its activity.

Examples

- Protamine neutralizes heparin.
- Chelating agents bind heavy metals.
- Antacids neutralize gastric acid.

5. Pharmacokinetic Antagonism

Definition

One drug reduces the concentration of another by altering its absorption, distribution, metabolism, or excretion.

Examples

- Rifampicin induces hepatic enzymes and reduces the effectiveness of oral contraceptives.
- Cholestyramine decreases absorption of certain medications.

Dose–Response Curves

Competitive Antagonists

- Shift the dose-response curve to the right.
- Do not reduce the maximal response (Emax).

Noncompetitive Antagonists

- Reduce the maximum response (Emax).
- Increasing agonist concentration cannot restore the maximal effect.

Clinical Applications

Understanding agonists and antagonists assists clinicians in:

- Selecting appropriate drug therapy.
- Reversing drug overdose.
- Treating poisoning.
- Managing cardiovascular disease.
- Treating asthma and chronic obstructive pulmonary disease.
- Managing pain.
- Treating endocrine and neurological disorders.

Summary Table

Drug Type	Affinity	Efficacy	Example
Full agonist	Yes	High	Morphine
Partial agonist	Yes	Moderate	Buprenorphine
Inverse agonist	Yes	Negative	Certain H_1 antihistamines*
Competitive antagonist	Yes	None	Atropine
Noncompetitive antagonist	Yes	None	Phenoxybenzamine

*Many modern H_1 antihistamines are better described pharmacologically as inverse agonists because they stabilize the inactive receptor state.

Learning Objectives

After studying this chapter, you should be able to:

- Define agonists and antagonists.
- Differentiate between affinity and efficacy.
- Classify agonists and antagonists.
- Explain the differences between competitive and noncompetitive antagonism. Describe physiological, chemical, and pharmacokinetic antagonism.
- Apply these concepts to clinical pharmacology and therapeutic decision-making.

Key Points to Remember

- Agonists bind to receptors and activate them.
- Antagonists bind to receptors without activating them and block receptor stimulation.
- Affinity is the ability to bind to a receptor; efficacy is the ability to produce a biological response.
- Full agonists produce maximal effects; partial agonists produce submaximal effects even when all receptors are occupied.
- Competitive antagonists can be overcome by increasing agonist concentration. Noncompetitive antagonists reduce the maximum response and cannot be overcome by increasing agonist concentration.
- Physiological antagonism involves opposing effects through different receptors. Chemical antagonism results from direct chemical interaction between substances.
- Pharmacokinetic antagonism occurs when one drug alters the absorption, metabolism, distribution, or excretion of another.

Exam Pearls

- Affinity = Binding; Efficacy = Activation.
- Agonist: Has both affinity and efficacy.
- Antagonist: Has affinity but no efficacy.
- Full agonist: Produces the maximum biological response.
- Partial agonist: Produces less than the maximum response and may antagonize a full agonist.
- Competitive antagonist: Reversible; shifts the dose-response curve to the right without reducing Emax.
- Noncompetitive antagonist: Decreases Emax and cannot be overcome by increasing agonist concentration.
- Naloxone is a competitive opioid receptor antagonist used to reverse opioid overdose.
- Protamine chemically antagonizes heparin.
- Rifampicin can produce pharmacokinetic antagonism by inducing hepatic enzymes and reducing the effectiveness of drugs such as oral contraceptives.

Dose–Response Relationships

Introduction

The dose–response relationship is one of the fundamental principles of pharmacology. It describes the relationship between the amount of a drug administered (dose) or the concentration of the drug at its site of action and the magnitude of the biological or therapeutic response produced.

Understanding dose–response relationships enables healthcare professionals to determine the most appropriate drug dosage, compare the effectiveness of different medications, predict therapeutic and toxic effects, and make safe prescribing decisions.

Dose–response analysis is widely used in drug development, clinical trials, and routine patient care to establish drug efficacy, potency, and safety.

Definition

A dose–response relationship is the relationship between the dose (or concentration) of a drug and the magnitude of the biological response it produces.

In general:

Increasing the drug dose increases the response.
A maximum response is eventually reached, beyond which further dose increases do not produce additional therapeutic benefit but may increase the risk of adverse effects.

Importance of Dose–Response Relationships

Understanding dose–response relationships helps healthcare professionals to:

- Select the optimal drug dose.
- Compare the potency and efficacy of drugs.
- Predict therapeutic outcomes.
- Recognize toxic doses.
- Establish the therapeutic range.
- Evaluate new drugsduring clinicaldevelopment.

Types of Dose–Response Relationships

There are two principal types:

- Graded Dose–Response Relationship Quantal
- Dose–Response Relationship

1. Graded Dose–Response Relationship

Definition

A graded dose–response relationship describes the continuous increase in response produced by increasing doses of a drug in a single individual or isolated tissue.

Characteristics

- Response increases progressively with dose.
- Maximum response (Emax) is eventually reached.
- Used to evaluate potency and efficacy

Examples

- Reduction in blood pressure after increasing doses of an antihypertensive drug.
- Bronchodilation after increasing doses of salbutamol.
- Progressive pain relief with increasing doses of morphine.

Components of a Graded Dose–Response Curve

A typical graded dose–response curve demonstrates:

1. Threshold Dose

The smallest dose that produces a measurable biological response.

2. Linear (Therapeutic) Portion

Within this range:

- Increasing the dose results in a proportional increase in response.
- This is the most useful range for clinical dosing.

3. Maximum Effect (Emax)

The greatest response a drug can produce.

Increasing the dose beyond Emax does not increase therapeutic benefit but may increase toxicity.

4. Plateau Phase

The portion of the curve where additional dose increases produce no further increase in effect because all available receptors or physiological mechanisms have been fully activated.

2. Quantal Dose–Response Relationship

Definition

A quantal dose–response relationship describes the percentage of a population that exhibits a predefined (all-or-none) response at different doses of a drug.

Each individual either:

- Responds, or
- Does not respond.

Uses

- Determining effective doses.
- Determining toxic doses.
- Determining lethal doses (in experimental studies). Evaluating drug safety.

Examples

- Percentage of patients achieving seizure control.
- Percentage of patients experiencing sleep after a sedative.
- Percentage of patients developing a particular adverse effect.

Potency

Definition

Potency refers to the amount of drug required to produce a specified effect.

A more potent drug requires a smaller dose to produce the same effect as a less potent drug.

Clinical Importance

- Determines the dose required.
- Does not indicate therapeutic superiority.

Example

Drug A produces pain relief at 5 mg, whereas Drug B requires 50 mg to produce the same degree of pain relief.

Drug A is more potent, but both drugs may be equally effective if they achieve the same maximum response.

- **Ef ficacy**

- **Definition**

- Efficacy (Intrinsic Activity) is the maximum effect that a drug can produce regardless of dose.

- **Clinical Importance**

- More important than potency when selecting therapy.
- Determines the greatest possible therapeutic benefit.

Example

Morphine has greater efficacy than codeine for severe pain because it produces a higher maximal analgesic effect.

EC_{50} (Median Effective Concentration)

Definition

EC_{50} is the concentration (or dose) of a drug that produces 50% of its maximal effect (Emax).

Significance

- Lower EC_{50} indicates greater potency.
- Frequently usedtocompare drugs.

ED_{50} (Median Effective Dose)

Definition

ED_{50} is the dose that produces the desired therapeutic effect in 50% of a population.

Used primarily in quantaldose–response studies.

TD_{50} (Median Toxic Dose)

Thedosethatproducesatoxiceffect in 50% of a population.

LD_{50} (Median Lethal Dose)

The dose that causes death in 50% of experimental animals.

Note: LD_{50} is used in preclinical research and is not determined in humans for ethical reasons.

Therapeutic Window

Definition

The therapeutic window is the range of drug concentrations between the minimum effective concentration (MEC) and the minimum toxic concentration (MTC).

Within this range:

- Therapeutic effects are achieved.
- Toxicity is minimized.

Drugs with a narrow therapeutic window require close monitoring.

Examples

- Digoxin
- Lithium
- Warfarin
- Theophylline

Factors Affecting the Dose–Response Relationship

Drug response varies among individuals because of differences in:

- Age
- Body weight
- Sex
- Genetics
- Disease states
- Liver function
- Kidney function
- Pregnancy
- Drug interactions
- Receptor sensitivity
- Tolerance

Clinical Applications

Dose–response relationships are essential for:

- Determining initial drug doses.
- Adjusting maintenance therapy.
- Comparing new medications.
- Monitoring drugs with narrow therapeutic windows.
- Avoiding toxicity.
- Individualizing patient treatment.

Summary Table

Term	Definition	Clinical Importance
Graded response	Continuous increase in response with dose	Determines potency and efficacy
Quantal response	All-or-none response in a population	Determines ED_{50}, TD_{50}
Potency	Dose required to produce an effect	Lower dose needed for the same effect
Efficacy	Maximum achievable effect	Determines therapeutic benefit
EC_{50}	Concentration producing 50% of Emax	Measures potency
ED_{50}	Effective dose in 50% of a population	Used in population studies
Therapeutic window	Range between effective and toxic concentrations	Guide safe dosing

Learning Objectives

After studying this chapter, you should be able to:

- Define dose–response relationships.
- Distinguish between graded and quantal dose–response curves.
- Explain potency and efficacy.
- Define EC_{50}, ED_{50}, TD_{50}, and LD_{50}.
- Describe the therapeutic window and its clinical significance.
- Apply dose–response principles to safe and effective drug therapy.

Key Points to Remember

- The dose–response relationship describes how drug dose influences biological response.
- Graded dose–response curves evaluate responses in individuals and are used to determine potency and efficacy.
- Quantal dose–response curves assess all-or-none responses in populations and are used to determine ED_{50} and TD_{50}.
- Potency refers to the amount of drug needed to produce a given effect.
- Efficacy refers to the maximum effect a drug can produce.
- EC_{50} is the concentration producing 50% of the maximal effect.
- The therapeutic window is the concentration range that provides efficacy with minimal toxicity.
- Drugs with a narrow therapeutic window require careful dosing and therapeutic monitoring.

Exam Pearls

- Potency = Dose required to produce an effect.
- Efficacy = Maximum effect a drug can produce.
- A more potent drug is not necessarily more effective.
- EC_{50} is inversely related to potency: the lower the EC_{50}, the greater the potency.
- ED_{50} is the dose effective in 50% of a population.
- TD_{50} is the dose producing toxicity in 50% of a population.
- LD_{50} is used only in experimental animal studies.
- The therapeutic window lies between the minimum effective concentration (MEC) and the minimum toxic concentration (MTC).
- Digoxin, lithium, warfarin, and theophylline are classic examples of drugs with a narrow therapeutic window requiring close monitoring.

Potency and Efficacy

Introduction

Potency and efficacy are two fundamental pharmacological concepts used to evaluate and compare the effects of drugs. Although these terms are often used together, they describe different characteristics of drug action.

Potency refers to the amount of a drug required to produce a specific effect, whereas efficacy refers to the maximum effect that a drug can produce regardless of dose. Understanding the distinction between potency and efficacy is essential for selecting appropriate medications, determining drug dosages, and interpreting dose–response relationships.

In clinical practice, efficacy is generally more important than potency because the primary goal is to achieve the desired therapeutic outcome safely and effectively.

Definitions

Potency

Potency is the amount (dose or concentration) of a drug required to produce a specified biological effect.

A highly potent drug produces the desired effect at a lower dose than a less potent drug.

Ef ficacy

Efficacy (Intrinsic Activity) is the maximum biological or therapeutic effect that a drug can produce after binding to its receptor.

Efficacy reflects the drug's ability to activate receptors and generate a response.

Potency versus Efficacy

Although related, potency and efficacy describe different aspects of drug action.

Feature	Potency	Efficacy
Definition	Dose required to produce a given effect	Maximum effect a drug can produce
Determined by	EC_{50} or ED_{50}	Maximum response (Emax)
Clinical Importance	Determines dosage	Determines therapeutic benefit
Influenced by	Affinity for receptor, pharmacokinetics	Intrinsic activity of the drug
Can be increased by higher dose?	No	Limited by the drug's maximal effect

Potency

Characteristics

A more potent drug:

- Requires a smaller dose.
- Has a lower EC_{50} or ED_{50}.
- Does not necessarily produce a greater therapeutic effect.

Example

Drug A produces pain relief at 5 mg, whereas Drug B requires 50 mg to produce the same level of pain relief.

Drug A is 10 times more potent than Drug B.

If both drugs relieve pain equally well, they have the same efficacy.

Factors Affecting Potency

Potency is influenced by:

- Drug affinity for receptors
- Drug absorption
- Distribution
- Metabolism
- Elimination
- Receptor sensitivity
- Drug formulation

Ef ficacy

Characteristics

A highly efficacious drug:

- Produces a greater maximum response.
- Is capable of treating more severe disease when appropriate.
- Cannot exceed its own maximal effect regardless of dose.

Increasing the dose beyond the maximal response increases the likelihood of adverseeffectswithoutimprovingtherapeutic benefit.

Factors Affecting Efficacy

Efficacy depends on:

- Intrinsic activity of the drug
- Number of available receptors
- Functional capacity of target tissues
- Disease severity
- Presence of receptor abnormalities

Potency and Dose–Response Curves

Both potency and efficacy can be evaluated using graded dose–response curves.

Potency

A more potent drug has its dose–response curve shifted to the left, indicating that a lower dose is needed to produce the same effect.

Ef ficacy

Amoreefficaciousdrugreaches a higher maximum response (Emax).

EC_{50} and Potency

Definition

EC_{50} (Median Effective Concentration) is the concentration of a drug that produces 50% of its maximal effect.

Interpretation

- Lower EC_{50} = Higher potency
- Higher EC_{50} = Lower potency

Emax and Efficacy

Emax represents the greatest response a drug can produce.

Two drugs may have:

- Different potencies
- The same efficacy

or

- Similar potencies
- Different efficacies

Full Agonists and Partial Agonists

The concepts of potency and efficacy are closely related to agonist activity.

Full Agonists

- Produce the maximal response.
- Have high efficacy.

Examples

- Morphine
- Epinephrine
- Salbutamol

Partial Agonists

- Produce less than the maximal response even when all receptors are occupied.
- Have lower efficacy than full agonists.

Examples

- Buprenorphine
- Aripiprazole
- Pindolol

Clinical Examples

Example 1: Morphine vs Codeine

Feature	Morphine	Codeine
Potency	Higher	Lower
Efficacy	Higher	Lower

Morphine is both more potent and more efficacious than codeine for the treatment of severe pain.

Example 2: Fentanyl vs Morphine

Feature	Fentanyl	Morphine
Potency	Much higher	Lower
Efficacy	Similar	Similar

Fentanyl requires a much smaller dose to produce analgesia but has a maximal analgesic effect comparable to morphine.

Example 3: Hydrochlorothiazide vs Furosemide

Furosemide is generally more efficacious than hydrochlorothiazide because it produces a greater maximal diuretic effect, especially in patients with significant edema.

Clinical Importance

Understanding potency and efficacy helps clinicians to:

- Select appropriate medications.
- Determine starting doses.
- Adjust maintenance therapy.
- Avoid toxicity.
- Compare therapeutic alternatives.
- Interpret clinical trials.
- Individualizepatient treatment.

Common Misconceptions

"More potent means better."

Incorrect.

A more potent drug simply requires a smaller dose.

It is not necessarily more effective clinically.

"A higher dose always produces a better response."

Incorrect.

Once the maximal response (Emax) has been reached, increasing the dose only increases the risk of adverse effects.

Summary Table

Characteristic	Potency	Efficacy
Definition	Amount of drug required for an effect	Maximum effect achievable
Determined by	EC_{50} or ED_{50}	Emax
Reflects	Drug strength	Therapeutic capability
More clinically important?	No	Yes
Increased dose changes it?	No	No

Learning Objectives

After studying this chapter, you should be able to:

Define potency and efficacy.
Differentiate between potency and efficacy.
Explain the relationship between EC_{50}, Emax, potency, and efficacy.
Compare full agonists and partial agonists based on efficacy.
Apply these concepts to rational drug selection and dosing.

Key Points to Remember

- Potency refers to the dose required to produce a given effect.
- Efficacy refers to the maximum effect a drug can produce.
- A more potent drug requires a lower dose, but is not necessarily more effective.
- Efficacy is generally more important than potency in clinical practice because it determines the greatest therapeutic benefit.
- EC_{50} is used to compare potency; a lower EC_{50} indicates greater potency.
- Emax reflects efficacy and represents the maximal achievable response.
- Full agonists have higher efficacy than partial agonists.

Exam Pearls

- Potency = Dose required to produce an effect.
- Efficacy = Maximum achievable effect (Emax).
- Lower EC_{50} = Greater potency.
- Higher Emax = Greater efficacy.
- Potency affects dose selection, whereas efficacy determines therapeutic benefit.
- A more potent drug is not necessarily superior to a less potent drug if both achieve the same maximal therapeutic effect.
- Full agonists have greater efficacy than partial agonists.
- Increasing the dose beyond Emax does not improve therapeutic benefit but does increase the risk of adverse effects.
- Fentanyl is much more potent than morphine, but both can achieve similar maximal analgesic effects.

Therapeutic Index

Introduction

The Therapeutic Index (TI) is an important measure of drug safety. It compares the dose of a drug that produces the desired therapeutic effect with the dose that causes toxicity. The therapeutic index helps healthcare professionals evaluate the safety margin of medications and determine the need for careful dose adjustment and therapeutic drug monitoring.

Drugs with a wide therapeutic index are generally considered safer because there is a large difference between effective and toxic doses. In contrast, drugs with a narrow therapeutic index require close monitoring since small changes in dose or blood concentration may result in toxicity or treatment failure.

Understanding the therapeutic index is essential for safe prescribing, preventing adverse drug reactions, and optimizing patient outcomes.

Definition

The Therapeutic Index (TI) is the ratio of the median toxic dose (TD_{50}) to the median effective dose (ED_{50}).

Formula

[
\boxed{\textbf{Therapeutic Index (TI) = \frac{TD_{50}}{ED_{50}}}}
]

Where:

- ED_{50} (Median Effective Dose): The dose that produces the desired therapeutic effect in 50% of the population.
- TD_{50} (Median Toxic Dose): The dose that produces toxic effects in 50% of the population.

In experimental animal studies, the Median Lethal Dose (LD_{50}) may be used instead of TD_{50}:

[

\boxed{\textbf{TI = \frac{LD_{50}}{ED_{50}}}}

]

Note: LD_{50} is not determined in humans for ethical reasons.

Formula

[
\boxed{\textbf{Therapeutic Index (TI) = \frac{TD_{50}}{ED_{50}}}}
]

- Where:
- ED_{50} (Median Effective Dose): The dose that produces the desired therapeutic effect in 50% of the population.
- TD_{50} (Median Toxic Dose): The dose that produces toxic effects in 50% of the population.

In experimental animal studies, the Median Lethal Dose (LD_{50}) may be used instead of TD_{50}:

[

\boxed{\textbf{TI = \frac{LD_{50}}{ED_{50}}}}

]

Note: LD_{50} is not determined in humans for ethical reasons.

Interpretation of the Therapeutic Index

The therapeutic index reflects the relative safety of a drug.

High Therapeutic Index

A high TI indicates:

- Wide margin of safety.
- Toxicity occurs only at doses much higher than therapeutic doses.
- Less intensive monitoring is generally required.

Low Therapeutic Index

A low TI indicates:

- Narrow margin of safety.
- Small increases in dose may cause toxicity.
- Careful dosing and therapeutic drug monitoring are often necessary.

Examples

Drug A

- ED_{50} = 10 mg
- TD_{50} = 200 mg

$$TI = \frac{200}{10} = 20$$

Interpretation: Drug A has a relatively wide therapeutic index and is generally considered safer.

Drug B

- ED_{50} = 10 mg
- TD_{50} = 20 mg

$$TI = \frac{20}{10} = 2$$

Interpretation: Drug B has a narrow therapeutic index and requires close monitoring.

Therapeutic Window

The therapeutic window (or therapeutic range) is the range of drug concentrations between the Minimum Effective Concentration (MEC) and the Minimum Toxic Concentration (MTC).

Within the therapeutic window:

- Desired therapeutic effects are achieved.
- Toxic effects are minimized.

Unlike the therapeutic index, which is a numerical ratio, the therapeutic window refers to the clinically useful concentration range in an individual patient.

Therapeutic Index versus Therapeutic Window

Feature	**Therapeutic Index**	**Therapeutic Window**
Definition	Ratio of toxic dosetoeffectivedose	Range of safe plasma drug concentrations
Expression	Numerical ratio (TD_{50}/ED_{50})	Concentration range (MEC to MTC)
Purpose	Estimates drug safety	Guides clinical dosing and monitoring
Clinical Use	Drug comparison	Individual patient management

Narrow Therapeutic Index (NTI) Drugs

Drugs with a narrow therapeutic index require careful dose adjustment because small changes in dosage or plasma concentration may lead to significant toxicity or loss of efficacy.

Common examples include:

Drug	Major Toxicity
Digoxin	Cardiac arrhythmias
Warfarin	Bleeding
Lithium	Neurological toxicity
Theophylline	Cardiac arrhythmias, seizures
Phenytoin	Neurological toxicity
Tacrolimus	Nephrotoxicity, neurotoxicity
Cyclosporine	Nephrotoxicity
Carbamazepine	Neurological toxicity, hematologic adverse effects

Drugs with a Wide Therapeutic Index

These medications generally have a larger safety margin.

Examples include:

- Penicillins
- Cephalosporins
- Most proton pump inhibitors
- Many H_2-receptor antagonists

Although these drugs are relatively safe, adverse effects and contraindications must still be considered.

Factors Affecting the Therapeutic Index

Several patient-related and drug-related factors influence the effective and toxic dose of medications.

These include:

- Age
- Body weight
- Genetic variation
- Liver disease
- Kidney disease
- Drug interactions
- Pregnancy
- Plasma protein binding
- Disease severity
- Medication adherence

Therapeutic Drug Monitoring (TDM)

Therapeutic Drug Monitoring (TDM) is the measurement of plasma drug concentrations to ensure that drug levels remain within the therapeutic window.

TDM is especially useful for drugs with:

- Narrow therapeutic index
- Significant pharmacokinetic variability
- Poor correlation between dose and plasma concentration

Common drugs requiring TDM include:

- Digoxin
- Lithium
- Phenytoin
- Vancomycin
- Aminoglycosides
- Tacrolimus
- Cyclosporine

Clinical Importance

Knowledge of the therapeutic index helps clinicians to:

- Select safer medications.
- Determine appropriate dosage regimens.
- Adjust doses in renal or hepatic impairment.
- Prevent drug toxicity.
- Monitor high-risk medications.
- Improve patient safety.

Limitations of the Therapeutic Index

Although useful, the therapeutic index has several limitations:

- Based on population averages rather than individual patients.
- Does not account for individual variability in drug response.
- Does not reflect differences in pharmacokinetics or pharmacodynamics.
- The therapeutic window is often more useful in day-to-day clinical practice.

Summary Table

Term	Definition	Clinical Importance
Therapeutic Index (TI)	$TD_{50} \div ED_{50}$	Estimates drug safety
ED_{50}	Effective dose in 50% of a population	Measures drug effectiveness
TD_{50}	Toxic dose in 50% of a population	Measures drug toxicity
Therapeutic Window	Range between MEC and MTC	Guides safe dosing
Therapeutic Drug Monitoring	Measurement of plasma drug levels	Prevents toxicity and treatment failure

Learning Objectives

After studying this chapter, you should be able to:

- Define the therapeutic index.
- Calculate the therapeutic index using ED_{50} and TD_{50}.
- Differentiate between the therapeutic index and the therapeutic window.
- Identify drugs with narrow therapeutic indices.
- Explain the role of therapeutic drug monitoring in clinical practice.
- Applytherapeutic indexconcepts to rational prescribing and patient safety.

Key Points to Remember

- The Therapeutic Index (TI) is a measure of drug safety and is calculated as $TD_{50} \div ED_{50}$.
- A high therapeutic index indicates a wide margin of safety.
- A low therapeutic index indicates a narrow margin of safety and requires careful monitoring.
- The therapeutic window is the concentration range between the Minimum Effective Concentration (MEC) and the Minimum Toxic Concentration (MTC).
- Drugs with a narrow therapeutic index often require therapeutic drug monitoring (TDM).
- Individual patient factors can significantly influence drug safety and therapeutic response.

Exam Pearls

- Therapeutic Index (TI) = $TD_{50} \div ED_{50}$.
- Higher TI = Greater drug safety.
- Lower TI = Greater risk of toxicity.
- Therapeutic window refers to the plasma concentration range between MEC and MTC.
- Digoxin, warfarin, lithium, phenytoin, theophylline, tacrolimus, and cyclosporine are classic narrow therapeutic index drugs.
- Therapeutic Drug Monitoring (TDM) is commonly used for drugs with narrow therapeutic indices to optimize efficacy while minimizing toxicity.
- LD_{50} is used in animal studies only and is not determined in humans.
- The therapeutic window is often more clinically useful than the therapeutic index for guiding individualized patient care.

Drug Selectivity

Introduction

Drug selectivity is the ability of a drug to act preferentially on a specific receptor, enzyme, ion channel, transporter, or tissue at therapeutic doses while producing minimal effects on other targets. Drug selectivity is one of the most important principles in pharmacology because it influences a drug's efficacy, safety, and adverse effect profile.

Most drugs are selective rather than specific. This means they preferentially interact with one target but may affect additional targets, especially at higher doses. Understanding drug selectivity helps healthcare professionals choose appropriate medications, predict adverse effects, and optimize patient care.

Definition

Drug selectivity is the preferential action of a drug on one molecular target or tissue over others at clinically relevant concentrations.

A selective drug produces its desired therapeutic effect primarily by acting on its intended target while minimizing effects on other receptors or organs.

Drug Selectivity versus Drug Specificity

Although the terms are sometimes used interchangeably, they have different meanings.

Feature	Drug Selectivity	Drug Specificity
Definition	Preference for one target over others	Acts only on one target
Clinical Reality	Common	Rare
Dose Dependent	Yes	Usually considered absolute
Example	Atenolol preferentially blocks β_1 receptors	Very few drugs are truly specific

Important Point

Virtually no drug is completely specific. Nearly all medications become less selective as the dose increases.

Basis of Drug Selectivity

Drug selectivity depends on several factors, including:

- Receptor affinity
- Receptor subtype distribution
- Drug concentration
- Tissue sensitivity
- Pharmacokinetic properties
- Route of administration
- Genetic variation

Mechanisms of Drug Selectivity

Drug selectivity may result from preferential interaction with:

1. Receptor Subtypes

Many receptors exist as multiple subtypes.

Examples

Drug	Selective Target	Clinical Effect
Atenolol	β_1-Adrenergic receptor	Lowers heart rate and blood pressure
Salbutamol	β_2-Adrenergic receptor	Bronchodilation
Tamsulosin	α_1A-Adrenergic receptor	Relieves urinary obstruction in benign prostatic hyperplasia
Mirabegron	β_3-Adrenergic receptor	Treats overactive bladder

2. Tissue Selectivity

Some drugs preferentially accumulate or act in certain tissues.

Examples

Drug	Tissue Preference
Bisphosphonates	Bone
Levothyroxine	Most body tissues via thyroid hormone receptors
Inhaled corticosteroids	Airways
Topical corticosteroids	Skin

3. Enzyme Selectivity

Some drugs selectively inhibit specific enzymes.

Examples

Drug	Selective Enzyme
Celecoxib	Cyclooxygenase-2 (COX-2)
Sildenafil	Phosphodiesterase type 5 (PDE-5)
Allopurinol	Xanthine oxidase
Donepezil	Acetylcholinesterase

4. Transporter Selectivity

Certain drugs selectively inhibit transport proteins.

Examples

Drug	Target
Fluoxetine	Serotonin transporter (SERT)
Empagliflozin	Sodium-glucose cotransporter 2 (SGLT2)
Digoxin	Na^+/K^+-ATPase

Dose-Dependent Loss of Selectivity

Drug selectivity decreases as the dose increases.

At therapeutic doses:

- The drug mainly affects its preferred target.

At higher doses:

- Additional receptors become occupied.
- Off-target effects increase.
- Adverse reactions become more common.

Example

Salbutamol

Low doses:

- Primarily stimulates β_2 receptors.
- Produces bronchodilation.

High doses:

- May stimulate β_1 receptors.
- Can cause tachycardia and palpitations.

Clinical Examples of Drug Selectivity

Beta-Adrenergic Blockers

Atenolol

- Selective β_1 blocker.
- Mainly affects the heart.
- Lower risk of bronchoconstriction than nonselective beta blockers.

Propranolol

- Nonselective β blocker.
- Blocks both β_1 and β_2 receptors.
- Mayprecipitate bronchospasminsusceptible individuals.

Cyclooxygenase Inhibitors

Celecoxib

- Selectively inhibits COX-2.
- Provides anti-inflammatory effects.
- Lower risk of gastrointestinal ulceration than traditional nonselective NSAIDs.

Ibuprofen

- Nonselective COX inhibitor.
- Inhibits both COX-1 and COX-2.

Alpha-Adrenergic Blockers

Tamsulosin

- Selective α_1A antagonist.
- Relaxes smooth muscle in the prostate and bladder neck.
- Produces less systemic hypotension than nonselective α_1 blockers.

Advantages of Drug Selectivity

Selective drugs may offer:

- Greater therapeutic efficacy
- Reduced adverse effects
- Improved patient safety
- Better tolerability
- More targeted therapy
- Improved patient adherence

Limitations of Drug Selectivity

Despite its advantages, selectivity has limitations.

- No drug is absolutely selective.
- Selectivity decreases with increasing dose.
- Disease states may alter receptor expression.
- Genetic variation can affect drug response.
- Drug interactions may modify selectivity.

Factors Affecting Drug Selectivity

Drug selectivity may be influenced by:

- Dose
- Age
- Genetic polymorphisms
- Liver disease
- Kidney disease
- Drug interactions
- Route of administration
- Receptor density
- Disease-related receptor changes

Clinical Importance

Understandingdrugselectivityhelps clinicians to:

- Choose safer medications.
- Reduce adverse drug reactions.
- Improve therapeutic outcomes.
- Select appropriate receptor-specific therapy.
- Individualizetreatment for patients with comorbid conditions.

Summary Table

Type of Selectivity	Example
Receptor selectivity	Atenolol (β_1), Salbutamol (β_2)
Tissue selectivity	Bisphosphonates (bone), Inhaled corticosteroids (airways)
Enzyme selectivity	Celecoxib (COX-2), Sildenafil (PDE-5)
Transporter selectivity	Fluoxetine (SERT), Empagliflozin (SGLT2)

Learning Objectives

After studying this chapter, you should be able to:

- Define drug selectivity.
- Differentiate between selectivity and specificity.
- Describe the mechanisms responsible for drug selectivity.
- Explain how drug dose influences selectivity.
- Apply the principles of drug selectivity to clinical pharmacology and therapeutic decision-making.

Key Points to Remember

- Drug selectivity is the preferential action of a drug on one receptor, enzyme, transporter, ion channel, or tissue.
- Most drugs are selective, not specific.
- Drug selectivity is dose dependent and generally decreases as the dose increases.
- Selective drugs often produce fewer adverse effects than nonselective drugs.
- Selectivity may involve receptor subtype, enzyme, transporter, or tissue preference.
- Genetic factors, disease states, and pharmacokinetics can influence drug selectivity.

Exam Pearls

- Selectivity ≠ Specificity. Virtually no drug is completely specific.
- Higher doses reduce selectivity and increase the likelihood of off-target adverse effects.
- Atenolol is relatively β_1-selective, whereas propranolol blocks both β_1 and β_2 receptors.
- Salbutamol selectively stimulates β_2 receptors at therapeutic doses but may cause tachycardia at higher doses due to loss of selectivity.
- Celecoxib selectively inhibits COX-2, resulting in less gastrointestinal toxicity than many nonselective NSAIDs.
- Tamsulosin selectively blocks α_1A receptors, improving urinary symptoms in benign prostatic hyperplasia with less orthostatic hypotension.
- Sildenafil selectively inhibits PDE-5, while fluoxetine selectively inhibits the serotonin transporter (SERT).
- Drug selectivity improves therapeutic precision but does not eliminate the risk of adverse effects.

Adverse Drug Reactions (ADRs)

Introduction

Drugs are intended to prevent, diagnose, or treat diseases; however, they may also produce undesirable or harmful effects in addition to their intended therapeutic actions. These unwanted effects are known as Adverse Drug Reactions (ADRs). ADRs are a major cause of patient morbidity, hospitalization, prolonged hospital stay, increased healthcare costs, and, in severe cases, mortality.

Healthcare professionals must be able to recognize, prevent, diagnose, and manage ADRs to ensure safe and effective pharmacotherapy. A thorough understanding of ADRs is essential for rational prescribing, patient counseling, and pharmacovigilance.

Definition

The World Health Organization (WHO) defines an Adverse Drug Reaction (ADR) as:

"A response to a drug that is noxious, unintended, and occurs at doses normally used in humans for the prophylaxis, diagnosis, treatment of disease, or modification of physiological function."

This definition excludes poisoning, overdose, medication errors, and drug abuse.

Adverse Drug Reaction versus Side Effect

Although often used interchangeably, these terms have different meanings.

Feature	Adverse Drug Reaction	Side Effect
Definition	Harmful and unintended response to a drug	Predictable secondary effect that may or may not
Severity	Usually clinically significant	Often mild
Desirable?	No	Occasionally beneficial
Example	Anaphylaxis after penicillin	Drowsiness with first-generation antihistamines

Classification of Adverse Drug Reactions

The traditional classification categorizes ADRs into six major types.

Type A (Augmented)

Characteristics

- Dose dependent
- Predictable
- Related to the known pharmacological action
- Common
- Usually preventable

Type A reactions account for approximately 70–80% of all ADRs.

Examples

Drug	ADR
Insulin	Hypoglycemia
Warfarin	Bleeding
Opioids	Respiratory depression
Antihypertensive drugs	Hypotension
NSAIDs	Gastric irritation and bleeding

Type B (Bizarre)

Characteristics

- Dose independent
- Unpredictable
- Not related to normal pharmacological action
- Often immune-mediated or genetically determined
- Rare but potentially life-threatening

Examples

Drug	ADR
Penicillin	Anaphylaxis
Carbamazepine	Stevens–Johnson syndrome
Chloramphenicol	Aplastic anemia
Sulfonamides	Severe hypersensitivity reactions

Type C (Chronic)

Characteristics

- Related to long-term drug use
- Develop gradually
- Often dose and duration dependent

Examples

Drug	ADR
Corticosteroids	Osteoporosis, adrenal suppression
Antipsychotics	Tardive dyskinesia
Proton pump inhibitors	Vitamin B_{12} deficiency (with prolonged use)

Type D (Delayed)

Characteristics

- Occur months or years after exposure
- Delayed onset

Examples

Drug	ADR
Alkylating anticancer agents	Secondary malignancies
Diethylstilbestrol (DES)	Vaginal clear cell carcinoma in exposed offspring
Radiation-sensitizingdrugs	Late tissue damage

Type E (End-of-Use)

Characteristics

- Occur after sudden discontinuation of therapy
- Withdrawal or rebound effects

Examples

Drug	ADR
Corticosteroids	Acute adrenal insufficiency
Clonidine	Rebound hypertension
Beta blockers	Rebound tachycardia or angina
Benzodiazepines	Withdrawal seizures and anxiety

Type F (Failure of Therapy)

Characteristics

- Unexpected failure of therapeutic effect
- Often due to drug interactions, resistance, poor adherence, or inadequate dosage

Examples

Drug	**ADR**
Antibiotics	Antimicrobial resistance
Oral contraceptives	Reduced effectiveness due to enzyme-inducing drugs
Antiepileptic drugs	Breakthrough seizures

Common Causes of ADRs

ADRs may result from:

- Excessive dosage
- Drug interactions
- Polypharmacy
- Allergic reactions
- Genetic variations
- Organ dysfunction (renal or hepatic impairment)
- Inappropriate prescribing
- Poor medication adherence
- Advanced age
- Pediatric age group

Risk Factors for ADRs

Patients at increased risk include:

- Older adults
- Infants and children
- Pregnant women
- Patients with liver disease
- Patients with kidney disease
- Patients taking multiple medications
- Individuals with previous drug allergies
- Patients withmultiple chronic illnesses

Drug Allergy

A drug allergy is an immune-mediated adverse reaction that occurs after exposure to a drug.

Characteristics include:

- Usually not dose dependent
- Requires prior sensitization (except in rare situations)
- May become more severe with repeated exposure

Clinical Manifestations

- Urticaria
- Angioedema
- Anaphylaxis
- Drug rash
- Bronchospasm
- Stevens–Johnson syndrome
- Toxic epidermal necrolysis

Drug Intolerance

Drug intolerance refers to an exaggerated response to the usual therapeutic dose of a drug.

Example

Severe tinnitus after a standard dose of aspirin.

Idiosyncratic Drug Reactions

These are uncommon, genetically determined abnormal responses that are unrelated to the drug's known pharmacological action.

Examples

- Hemolysis with primaquine in patients with glucose-6-phosphate dehydrogenase (G6PD) deficiency
- Malignant hyperthermia triggered by certain inhalational anesthetics and succinylcholineingenetically susceptible individuals

Drug Toxicity

Drug toxicity occurs when excessive drug concentrations cause harmful effects.

Causes include:

- Overdose
- Drug accumulation
- Impaired metabolism
- Impaired elimination
- Drug interactions

Examples

- Digoxin toxicity
- Acetaminophen overdose
- Lithium toxicity

Prevention of ADRs

Healthcare professionals can reduce ADRs by:

- Obtaining a complete medication history.
- Reviewing allergy history.
- Avoiding unnecessary polypharmacy.
- Prescribing the lowest effective dose.
- Adjusting doses for renal or hepatic impairment.
- Monitoring high-risk medications.
- Educating patients regarding proper medication use.
- Reporting serious ADRsthrough pharmacovigilance programs.

Pharmacovigilance

Pharmacovigilance is the science and activities related to the detection, assessment, understanding, prevention, and reporting of adverse drug reactions and other medication-related problems.

Its goals include:

- Improving patient safety.
- Identifying rare adverse effects.
- Monitoring newly approved medications.
- Updating prescribing information.
- Supporting regulatory decision-making.

Clinical Importance

Recognizing ADRsenablesclinicians to:

- Improve medication safety.
- Reduce preventable hospital admissions.
- Optimize drug therapy.
- Educate patients effectively.
- Identify high-risk individuals.
- Report seriousadverse events to pharmacovigilance systems.

Summary Table

Type	Description	Examples
Type A	Augmented, dose dependent, predictable	Hypoglycemia with insulin, bleeding with warfarin
Type B	Bizarre, dose independent, unpredictable	Penicillin anaphylaxis, Stevens–Johnson syndrome
Type C	Chronic	Osteoporosis from corticosteroids
Type D	Delayed	Secondary malignancies after chemotherapy
Type E	End-of-use (withdrawal)	Adrenal crisis after abrupt steroid withdrawal
Type F	Failure of therapy	Antibiotic resistance, contraceptive failure

Learning Objectives

Afterstudyingthis chapter,youshould be able to:

- Define adverse drug reactions.
- Differentiate ADRs from side effects.
- Classify ADRs according to the traditional Type A–F system.
- Identify risk factors for ADRs.
- Distinguish between drug allergy, intolerance, idiosyncratic reactions, and
- toxicity. Describe strategies for preventing and reporting ADRs.

Key Points to Remember

- An Adverse Drug Reaction (ADR) is a harmful, unintended response to a drug used at normal therapeutic doses.
- Type A reactions are dose dependent, predictable, and account for the majority of ADRs.
- Type B reactions are unpredictable and often immune-mediated or genetically determined.
- Long-term therapy may cause Type C reactions, whereas Type D reactions appear after a delayed period.
- Type E reactions occur after abrupt drug withdrawal.
- Type F reactions represent unexpected failure of therapy.
- Older adults, children, patients with renal or hepatic impairment, and those receiving multiple medications are at increased risk.
- Pharmacovigilance plays a critical role in identifying, preventing, and reporting ADRs.

Exam Pearls

- WHO Definition: ADRs occur at normal therapeutic doses and are harmful and unintended.
- Type A (Augmented): Predictable, dose dependent, and the most common type of ADR.
- Type B (Bizarre): Unpredictable, not dose dependent, often related to allergy or genetics.
- Penicillin may cause anaphylaxis, a classic Type B ADR.
- Warfarin commonly causes bleeding, a classic Type A ADR.
- Abrupt withdrawal of corticosteroids may lead to acute adrenal insufficiency (Type E).
- Drug allergy is immune-mediated, whereas drug intolerance is an exaggerated response to a normal dose.
- G6PD deficiency predisposes patients to hemolysis with oxidant drugs such as primaquine.
- Pharmacovigilance is essential for detecting rare and serious adverse drug reactions after medications are marketed.

Drug Safety

Introduction

Drug safety is a fundamental principle of pharmacology and clinical practice. It refers to the safe and appropriate use of medications to maximize therapeutic benefits while minimizing the risk of adverse effects, medication errors, toxicity, and drug interactions. Every medication has the potential to cause harm if used improperly; therefore, ensuring drug safety is a shared responsibility among physicians, pharmacists, nurses, and patients.

Safe medication use involves selecting the appropriate drug, prescribing the correct dose, choosing the proper route and duration of administration, monitoring therapeutic response, recognizing adverse drug reactions, and educating patients about the safe use of medications.

Drug safety is an essential component of patient safety, evidence-based prescribing, and quality healthcare.

Definition

Drug safety is the prevention, identification, assessment, and management of risks associated with the use of medications to ensure that their therapeutic benefits outweightheir potential harms.

Objectives of Drug Safety

The primary objectives of drug safety are to:

- Maximize therapeutic effectiveness.
- Minimize adverse drug reactions (ADRs).
- Prevent medication errors.
- Reduce drug toxicity.
- Avoid harmful drug interactions.
- Improve patient adherence.
- Enhance overall patient safety.

Principles of Safe Drug Use

Safe medication practice is based on several key principles.

1. Right Patient

Verify the patient's identity before administering any medication.

Methods include:

- Full name
- Date of birth
- Hospital identification number Identification wristband (hospital setting)

2. Right Drug

Ensure that the prescribed medication matches the patient's diagnosis and medical condition.

Always confirm:

- Generic and brand names
- Drug strength
- Dosage form
- Expiration date

3. Right Dose

Administer the correct dose based on:

- Age
- Body weight
- Body surface area (when appropriate)
- Kidney function
- Liver function
- Clinical condition

4. Right Route

Confirm the correct route of administration.

Examples include:

- Oral
- Intravenous
- Intramuscular
- Subcutaneous
- Topical Inhalational

5. Right Time

Administer medications at the prescribed time and appropriate intervals to maintain therapeutic druglevels.

6. Right Documentation

Accurately record:

- Drug administered
- Dose
- Time
- Route
- Patient response
- Any adverse effects

7. Right Reason

Ensurethateverymedication has a clear clinical indication.

8. Right Response

Monitor therapeutic effectiveness and observe for adverse reactions.

Medication Errors

A medication error is any preventable event that may lead to

inappropriate medication use or patient harm.

Medication errors may occur during:

- Prescribing
- Transcribing
- Dispensing
- Administration
- Monitoring

Common Causes of Medication Errors

- Illegible prescriptions
- Incorrect dosage calculations
- Similar drug names (look-alike/sound-alike medications)
- Polypharmacy
- Poor communication
- Inadequate patient education
- Failure to review allergies
- Failure to adjust doses in renal or hepatic impairment

Strategies to Prevent Medication Errors

Healthcare professionals should:

- Verify patient identity.
- Review allergies before prescribing.
- Use generic names whenever possible. Double-check high-risk medications.
- Avoid unsafe abbreviations.
- Reconcile medications during transitions of care. Educate patients regarding medication use.
- Use electronic prescribing systems when available.

High-Alert Medications

High-alertmedicationshaveanincreased risk of causing significant harm if used incorrectly.

Examples include:

Drug Class	**Examples**
Anticoagulants	Warfarin, Heparin
Insulin	All insulin preparations
Opioids	Morphine, Fentanyl
Chemotherapy drugs	Methotrexate, Cisplatin
Electrolytes	Potassium chloride (IV), Magnesium sulfate
Sedatives	Midazolam, Propofol

These medications require additional safeguards during prescribing, dispensing, and administration.

Medication Reconciliation

Medication reconciliation is the systematic process of comparing a patient's current medications with newly prescribed medications during transitions of care.

It helps prevent:

- Drug duplication
- Drug omissions
- Drug interactions
- Incorrect dosing

Medication reconciliation should be performed:

- On hospital admission
- During transfer between healthcare settings
- At hospital discharge
- During outpatient follow-up visits

Patient Education

Patient education plays a vital role in drug safety.

Patients should be instructed regarding:

- Drug name and purpose
- Correct dose
- Administration schedule
- Duration of therapy
- Possible adverse effects
- Drug interactions
- Storage conditions
- Missed-dose instructions
- When to seek medical attention

Safe Prescribing

Safe prescribing requires clinicians to:

- Confirm the diagnosis.
- Select the most appropriate drug.
- Review allergies.
- Assess kidney and liver function.
- Consider pregnancy and breastfeeding.
- Evaluate potential drug interactions.
- Use the lowest effective dose.
- Avoid unnecessary polypharmacy.

Safe Drug Administration

Healthcare professionals should:

- Follow the "Rights" of medication administration.
- Confirm patient identity.
- Use aseptic techniques when appropriate.
- Monitor for adverse effects.
- Document administration accurately.
- Report medication errors promptly.

Monitoring Drug Therapy

Drug therapy should be monitored by assessing:

- Therapeutic effectiveness
- Adverse drug reactions
- Laboratory investigations
- Vital signs
- Organ function
- Patient adherence

Examples of laboratory monitoring include:

- INR for warfarin
- Blood glucose for insulin
- Serum lithium concentration
- Serum digoxin concentration
- Serum creatinine for nephrotoxic drugs

Special Populations

Certain groups require extra attention because of altered pharmacokinetics and pharmacodynamics.

These include:

Older Adults

- Increased sensitivity to many drugs
- Reduced renal and hepatic function
- Higher risk of falls and ADRs

Children

- Weight-based dosing
- Immature organ function
- Increased risk of dosing errors

Pregnant Women

- Avoid teratogenic drugs
- Consider placental drug transfer
- Evaluate maternal and fetal risks and benefits

Patients with Kidney Disease

- Adjust doses of renally eliminated drugs
- Monitor kidney function
- Prevent drug accumulation

Patients with Liver Disease

- Reduce doses when hepatic metabolism is impaired
- Monitor liver function tests
- Avoid hepatotoxic medications when possible

Pharmacovigilance

Pharmacovigilance is the science of detecting, assessing, understanding, preventing, and reporting adverse drug reactions and other medication-related problems.

Its objectives include:

- Improving medication safety
- Detecting rare adverse reactions
- Monitoring newly marketed drugs
- Supporting regulatory decisions
- Protecting public health

Clinical Importance

Drug safety improves:

- Therapeutic outcomes
- Patient adherence
- Quality of care
- Medication effectiveness
- Prevention of avoidable adverse events
- Healthcare cost reduction

Summary Table

Principle	Purpose
Right patient	Prevent administration to the wrong patient
Right drug	Ensure correct medication selection Prevent
Right dose	underdosing and overdosing Ensure proper
Right route	drug delivery
Right time	Maintain therapeutic drug levels
Right documentation	Provide an accurate medical record Confirm
Right reason	appropriate indication
Right response	Assesseffectiveness and detect ADRs

Learning Objectives

After studying this chapter, you should be able to:

- Define drug safety.
- Describe the principles of safe medication use.
- Identify common causes of medication errors.
- Explain strategies to prevent medication errors.
- Discuss the role of medication reconciliation and patient education.
- Apply drug safety principles in clinical practice.

Key Points to Remember

- Drug safety aims to maximize therapeuticbenefits while minimizing medication-related harm.
- The Eight Rights of Medication Administration are: Right Patient, Right Drug, Right Dose, Right Route, Right Time, Right Documentation, Right Reason, and Right Response.
- Medication errors can occur during prescribing, dispensing, administration, or monitoring and are often preventable.
- High-alert medications, such as insulin, anticoagulants, opioids, chemotherapy drugs, and concentrated intravenous electrolytes, require additional safety precautions.
- Medication reconciliation helps prevent omissions, duplications, interactions, and dosing errors during transitions of care.
- Patient education is essential for improving medication adherence and reducing preventable adverse drug events.
- Older adults, children, pregnant women, and patients with renal or hepatic impairment require individualized dosing and closer monitoring.
- Pharmacovigilance contributes to identifying, evaluating, and preventing medication-related harm after drugs are marketed

Exam Pearls

- Drug safety focuses on ensuring that the benefits of drug therapy outweigh its risks.
- Remember the Eight Rights of Medication Administration: Patient, Drug, Dose, Route, Time, Documentation, Reason, and Response.
- Medication reconciliation should be performed at admission, transfer, discharge, and outpatient follow-up to reduce medication errors.
- High-alert medications include warfarin, heparin, insulin, opioids, chemotherapy agents, and concentrated IV potassium chloride.
- Older adults are at increased risk of adverse drug reactions because of reduced renal and hepatic function and polypharmacy.
- Children require weight-based dosing, while patients with renal or hepatic impairment often require dose adjustment.
- Warfarin therapy is monitored using the International Normalized Ratio (INR).
- Lithium, digoxin, aminoglycosides, and vancomycin commonly require therapeutic drug monitoring (TDM).
- Clear communication, accurate documentation, patient education, and prompt reporting of medication errors are essential components of safe medication practice.

Medication Errors

Introduction

Medication errors are among the most common preventable causes of patient harm in healthcare. They may occur at any stage of the medication-use process, including prescribing, transcribing, dispensing, preparing, administering, and monitoring medications. Medication errors can lead to adverse drug events, prolonged hospitalization, increased healthcare costs, permanent disability, or even death.

Most medication errors are preventable through standardized procedures, effective communication, proper patient identification, medication reconciliation, and adherence to established safety guidelines. Understanding the causes, types, prevention strategies, and reporting of medication errors is essential for all healthcare professionals.

Definition

The National Coordinating Council for Medication Error Reporting and Prevention (NCC MERP) defines a medication error as:

"Any preventable event that may cause or lead to inappropriate medication use or patient harm while the medication is in the control of the healthcare professional, patient, or consumer."

Medication errors may or may not result in patient harm.

Medication Error versus Adverse Drug Reaction

Although related, medication errors and adverse drug reactions are different.

Feature	Medication Error	Adverse DrugReaction(ADR)
Definition	Preventable mistake during medication use	Harmful, unintended response at normal dose
Preventable	Usually yes	Often not preventable
Cause	Human or systemerror	Drug-related biological response
Example	Administering the wrong dose	Penicillin-induced anaphylaxis

Stages of Medication Use

Medicationerrorsmayoccurduringanyof the following stages:

1. Prescribing
2. Transcribing
3. Dispensing
4. Preparing
5. Administering
6. Monitoring

Types of Medication Errors

1. Prescribing Errors

Errors occurring during drug selection or prescription writing.

Examples

- Wrong drug
- Incorrect dose
- Incorrect dosage form
- Wrong frequency
- Wrong route
- Failure to recognize drug allergy
- Failure to consider drug interactions
- Inappropriateprescribing in renal or hepatic impairment

2. Transcribing Errors

Errors made while transferring medication orders.

Examples

- Incorrect transcription of dose
- Omission of medications
- Misinterpretation of handwritten prescriptions
- Incorrect patient identification

Electronic prescribing systems have significantly reduced many transcribing errors.

3. Dispensing Errors

Errors occurring during medication preparation or dispensing by the pharmacy.

Examples

- Wrong medication dispensed
- Wrong strength
- Incorrect labeling
- Expired medication
- Wrong dosage form

4. Administration Errors

Errors occurring when medications are given to patients.

Examples

- Wrong patient
- Wrong medication
- Wrong dose
- Wrong route
- Wrong time
- Omitted dose
- Incorrect infusion rate

Administration errors are among the most common medication errors.

5. Monitoring Errors

Failure to appropriately monitor medication therapy.

Examples

- Failure to monitor INR in patients receiving warfarin
- Failure to monitor blood glucose in patients receiving insulin
- Failure to monitor serum lithium concentrations
- Failure to detect adverse drug reactions

Common Causes of Medication Errors

Medication errors usually result from multiple contributing factors.

These include:

- Illegible handwriting
- Similar drug names (look-alike/sound-alike medications)
- Similar packaging
- Incorrect dosage calculations
- Poor communication
- Fatigue
- Heavy workload
- Inadequate staffing
- Interruptions during medication preparation
- Inadequate training
- Polypharmacy
- Lack of medication reconciliation

High-Risk Situations

Medication errors are more likely in:

- Emergency departments
- Intensive care units
- Pediatric patients
- Older adults
- Patients receiving multiple medications
- Patients with renal or hepatic impairment
- Patients taking high-alert medications

High-Alert Medications

High-alert medications are drugs that carry a greater risk of causing significant harm if used incorrectly.

Examples include:

Drug Class	Examples
Anticoagulants	Warfarin, Heparin
Insulin	All insulin preparations
Opioids	Morphine, Fentanyl
Chemotherapy drugs	Methotrexate, Cisplatin
Intravenous electrolytes	Potassium chloride, Magnesium sulfate
Sedatives	Midazolam, Propofol

These medications require additional safeguards and independent verification whenever possible.

Prevention of Medication Errors

Medication errors can be reduced through systematic safety practices.

Safe Prescribing

- Use clear and complete prescriptions.
- Prefer generic drug names.
- Avoid unsafe abbreviations.
- Review allergies before prescribing.
- Check renal and hepatic function.
- Consider potential drug interactions.

Safe Dispensing

- Verify medication labels carefully.
- Double-check high-alert medications.
- Store look-alike/sound-alike drugs separately.
- Remove expired medications promptly.

Safe Administration

Follow the Eight Rights of Medication Administration:

1. Right patient
2. Right drug
3. Right dose
4. Right route
5. Right time
6. Right documentation
7. Right reason
8. Right response

Medication Reconciliation

Medication reconciliation involves comparing the patient's current medications with new medication orders to prevent:

- Drug omissions
- Duplicate therapy
- Drug interactions
- Incorrect dosages

Medication reconciliation should be performed:

- At hospital admission
- During transfers between healthcare settings
- At hospital discharge
- During outpatientfollow-up

Patient Education

Patients should understand:

- Drug name and purpose
- Correct dose
- Timing of administration
- Duration of treatment
- Possible adverse effects
- Missed-dose instructions
- When to seek medical attention

Educated patients are more likely to recognize and report medication-related problems.

Reporting Medication Errors

Healthcare professionals should report medication errors promptly to improve patient safety.

Reporting systems aim to:

- Identify contributing factors
- Prevent recurrence
- Improve healthcare systems
- Promote a culture of safety rather than blame

Near misses should also be reported because they provide valuable opportunities for system improvement.

Role of Technology

Modern healthcare systems use technology to reduce medication errors.

Examples include:

- Computerized provider order entry (CPOE)
- Electronic prescribing (e-prescribing)
- Barcode medication administration (BCMA)
- Clinical decision support systems (CDSS)
- Automated dispensing cabinets
- Smart infusion pumps

These technologies reduce—but do not eliminate—the risk of medication errors.

Clinical Importance

Preventing medication errors:

- Improves patient safety
- Reduces preventable adverse drug events
- Decreases hospital admissions
- Lowers healthcare costs
- Enhances patient confidence in healthcare services

Summary Table

Type of Error	Examples
Prescribing	Wrong drug, wrong dose, allergy overlooked
Transcribing	Incorrect transfer of medication orders
Dispensing	Wrong medication, incorrect labeling
Administration	Wrong patient, wrong route, wrong time
Monitoring	Failure to monitor INR, glucose, or serum drug levels

Learning Objectives

After studying this chapter, you should be able to:

- Define a medication error.
- Differentiate medication errors from adverse drug reactions.
- Identify the different types of medication errors.
- Recognize common causes and high-risk situations.
- Describe strategies to prevent medication errors.
- Explain the role of medication reconciliation, patient education, and reporting systems in improving medication safety.

Key Points to Remember

- A medication error is a preventable event that may lead to inappropriate medication use or patient harm.
- Medication errors can occur during prescribing, transcribing, dispensing, preparing, administering, or monitoring medications.
- Medication errors are different from adverse drug reactions (ADRs) because they are generally preventable.
- Administration errors are among the most frequently reported medication errors.
- Look-alike/sound-alike medications, poor communication, fatigue, and polypharmacy are common causes of medication errors.
- High-alert medications, such as insulin, anticoagulants, opioids, chemotherapy agents, and concentrated intravenous electrolytes, require additional safety precautions.
- Following the Eight Rights of Medication Administration helps reduce administration errors.
- Medication reconciliation is essential during transitions of care to prevent omissions, duplications, interactions, and dosing errors.
- Healthcare professionals should report medication errors and near misses to improve healthcare systems and patient safety.
- Technologies such as electronic prescribing, barcode medication administration, and clinical decision support systems significantly reduce—but do not eliminate—medication errors.

Exam Pearls

- Medication errors are preventable, whereas adverse drug reactions may occur despite correct medication use.
- The NCC MERP defines a medication error as any preventable event that may cause inappropriate medication use or patient harm.
- The most common stages for medication errors include prescribing, dispensing, administration, and monitoring.
- Administration errors frequently involve the wrong patient, wrong drug, wrong dose, wrong route, or wrong time.
- Insulin, warfarin, heparin, opioids, chemotherapy drugs, and intravenous potassium chloride are classic high-alert medications.
- The Eight Rights of Medication Administration are essential for preventing medication administration errors.
- Medication reconciliation should be performed at hospital admission, transfer, discharge, and outpatient follow-up.
- Electronic prescribing (e-prescribing), barcode medication administration (BCMA), computerized provider order entry (CPOE), and clinical decision support systems (CDSS) help reduce medication errors.
- Near misses should be reported because they identify system weaknesses and provide opportunities to improve patient safety.

Essential Medicines

Introduction

Essential medicines are medications that satisfy the priority healthcare needs of a population. They are selected based on their proven efficacy, safety, quality, and cost-effectiveness to ensure that the most important health conditions can be treated with available resources.

The concept of essential medicines was introduced by the World Health Organization (WHO) in 1977 to promote equitable access to safe, effective, and affordable medicines worldwide. Today, essential medicines are the cornerstone of national healthcare systems, primary healthcare programs, and universal health coverage.

Healthcare professionals should be familiar with the principles of essential medicines because they support rational prescribing, improve patient outcomes, reduce healthcare costs, and ensure the efficient use of limited healthcare resources.

Definition

According to the World Health Organization (WHO):
Essential medicines are those that satisfy the priority healthcare needs of a population. They should be:

- Available at all times.
- Available in adequate quantities.
- Available in appropriate dosage forms.
- Of assured quality.
- Affordable to individuals and healthcare systems.

Objectives of Essential Medicines

The primary objectives are to:

- Improve access to safe and effective medicines.
- Promote rational use of medicines.
- Reduce morbidity and mortality.
- Ensure equitable distribution of healthcare resources.
- Improve public health.
- Reduce healthcare costs.

Criteria for Selection of Essential Medicines

Medicines are selected based on several important criteria.

1. Public Health Relevance

Medicines should address diseases that impose a significant burden on the population.

Examples include:

- Hypertension
- Diabetes mellitus
- Tuberculosis
- Malaria
- HIV infection
- Asthma

2. Proven Efficacy

Medicines should have strong scientific evidence demonstrating clinical effectiveness .

Selection is based on:

- Clinical trials
- Systematic reviews
- Evidence-based guidelines

3. Safety

The benefits of the medicine should outweigh its risks when used appropriately.

Safety evaluation includes:

- Adverse drug reactions
- Contraindications
- Drug interactions
- Toxicity profile

4. Cost-Effectiveness

Medicines should provide the greatest health benefit at the lowest reasonable cost.

Cost-effectiveness considers:

- Drug acquisition cost
- Treatment success
- Reduction in hospitalization
- Long-term healthcare savings

5. Quality

Essential medicines must meet recognized standards of:

- Identity
- Purity
- Potency
- Stability Manufacturing quality

WHO Model List of Essential Medicines

The WHO Model List of Essential Medicines (EML) is updated periodically by the World Health Organization.

The list serves as a model for countries to develop their own national essential medicines lists based on local disease patterns and healthcare priorities.

The WHO Model List includes medicines for:

- Infectious diseases
- Cardiovascular diseases
- Endocrine disorders
- Respiratory diseases
- Gastrointestinal disorders
- Mental health conditions
- Cancer
- Emergency medicine
- Vaccinesand biologicalproducts

Categories of Essential Medicines

Essential medicines cover a broad range of therapeutic areas.

Examples include:

Therapeutic Category	Examples
Analgesics	Paracetamol, Morphine
Antibiotics	Amoxicillin, Ceftriaxone
Antihypertensives	Amlodipine, Enalapril
Antidiabetic drugs	Metformin, Insulin
Antiasthmatic drugs	Salbutamol
Antimalarials	Artemisinin-based combination therapies
Antiepileptic drugs	Sodium valproate, Carbamazepine
Vaccines	Measles, Polio, Hepatitis B
Emergency medicines	Epinephrine, Atropine

National Essential Medicines Lists

Many countries develop their own National Essential Medicines List (NEML) based on:

- Local disease prevalence
- National treatment guidelines
- Healthcare resources
- Availability of medicines
- Cost considerations

National listsare usuallyadaptedfromtheWHOModel List.

Benefits of Essential Medicines

Implementationofessentialmedicinesprogramsprovides numerous advantages.

These include:

- Improved access to treatment.
- Better patient outcomes.
- Rational prescribing.
- Reduced medication shortages.
- Improved quality of healthcare.
- Lower healthcare expenditure.
- Better inventory management.
- Increased availability oflifesavingmedications.

Rational Use of Essential Medicines

TheWorld Health Organization definesrationalmedicine use as:

"Patients receive medications appropriate to their clinical needs, in doses that meet their individual requirements, for an adequate period, and at the lowest cost to them and their community."

Rational prescribing requires:

- Correct diagnosis
- Appropriate drug selection
- Correct dose
- Appropriate route
- Appropriate duration
- Patient education
- Monitoring for efficacy and adverse effects

Challenges in Essential Medicines Programs

Common challenges include:

- Drug shortages
- Limited financial resources
- Counterfeit medicines
- Inadequate supply chains
- Poor prescribing practices
- Antimicrobial resistance
- Inadequate healthcare infrastructure

Role of Healthcare Professionals

Healthcare professionals contribute to the success of essential medicines programs

by:

- Prescribing according to evidence-based guidelines.
- Promoting rational drug use.
- Preventing unnecessary polypharmacy.
- Educating patients.
- Monitoring treatment outcomes.
- Reporting adverse drug reactions.
- Supporting antimicrobialstewardship.

Clinical Importance

Essential medicines improve healthcare by:

- Increasing access to effective treatments.
- Reducing preventable disease complications.
- Improving medication affordability.
- Supporting universal health coverage.
- Promoting evidence-based prescribing.
- Optimizing limited healthcare resources.

Summary Table

Principle	Description
Public health relevance	Addresses priority diseases
Proven efficacy	Supported by scientific evidence
Safety	Acceptable benefit-risk profile
Cost-effectiveness	Provides maximum health benefit at reasonable cost
Quality	Meets recognized manufacturing standards
Availability	Accessible in adequate quantities and dosage forms

Learning Objectives

After studying this chapter, you should be able to:

- Define essential medicines.
- Describe the objectives of the Essential Medicines Program.
- Explain the criteria used to select essential medicines.
- Discuss the role of the WHO Model List of Essential Medicines.
- Describe the principles of rational medicine use.
- Recognize the importance of essential medicines in improving public health.

Key Points to Remember

- Essential medicines satisfy the priority healthcare needs of a population.
- The concept was introduced by the World Health Organization (WHO) in 1977.
- Essential medicines should be available at all times, in adequate quantities, in appropriate dosage forms, with assured quality, and at affordable prices.
- Selection is based on public health relevance, efficacy, safety, quality, and cost-effectiveness.
- The WHO Model List of Essential Medicines serves as a guide for countries developing their own national essential medicines lists.
- National Essential Medicines Lists (NEMLs) are adapted to local disease patterns and healthcare priorities.
- Rational prescribing and the appropriate use of essential medicines improve patient outcomes and reduce healthcare costs.
- Healthcare professionals play a vital role in ensuring the safe, effective, and rational use ofessential medicines.

Exam Pearls

- WHO Definition: Essential medicines are those that satisfy the priority healthcare needs of a population.
- The WHO Model List of Essential Medicines was first introduced in 1977.
- Essential medicines are selected based on efficacy, safety, quality, cost-effectiveness, and public health relevance.
- Essential medicines should be continuously available in adequate quantities and appropriate dosage forms.
- The WHO Model List serves as a model, while each country develops its own National Essential Medicines List (NEML).
- Rational use of medicines means prescribing the right medicine, for the right patient, at the right dose, for the right duration, and at the lowest appropriate cost .
- Examples of commonly listed essential medicines include paracetamol, amoxicillin, metformin, insulin, salbutamol, amlodipine, morphine, and epinephrine.
- Essential medicines are a key component of primary healthcare, patient safety, and universal health coverage.
- Promoting the use of essential medicines improves access to treatment, enhances healthcare quality, and optimizes the use of limited healthcare resources.

Generic and Brand-Name Drugs

Introduction

Medications are commonly marketed under generic names and brand (trade) names. Understanding the differences between these two types of drug names is essential for healthcare professionals because it promotes rational prescribing, reduces medication errors, improves communication, and helps lower healthcare costs.
A generic drug contains the same active ingredient as its corresponding brand-name drug and is expected to have the same dosage form, strength, route of administration, quality, safety, efficacy, and therapeutic effect. Generic drugs are generally less expensive because manufacturers do not bear the initial costs of drug discovery and development.
Healthcare providers should understand when generic substitution is appropriate and recognize situations in which brand-name prescribing may be necessary.

Drug Nomenclature Review

A drug may have several different names during its development and marketing.

Type of Name	Description	Example (Paracetamol)
Chemical Name	Describes the chemical structure of the drug	N-(4- hydroxyphenyl)acetamide
Generic (Nonproprietary) Name	Official name assigned to the active ingradient	paracetamole (Acetomenophen)
Brand (Trade/Proprietary)	Name chosen by the manufacturer for marketing	Tylenol , panadol

Generic Drugs

Definition

A generic drug is a medication that contains the same active ingredient as the original brand-name drug and is approved to be bioequivalent to the brand-name product.

Generic drugs must demonstrate:

- The same active ingredient
- The same strength
- The same dosage form
- The same route of administration
- Comparable quality
- Bioequivalence
- Similar therapeutic effectiveness
- Comparablesafety profile

Brand-Name Drugs

Definition

A brand-name drug (also called a trade-name or proprietary drug) is the original medication developed and marketed by a pharmaceutical company under a registered trademark.

Brand-name drugs are protected by patents for a limited period, allowing the manufacturer exclusive marketing rights before generic versions become available.

Characteristics of Generic Drugs

Generic drugs:

- Contain the same active pharmaceutical ingredient (API).
- Are bioequivalent to the brand-name product.
- Produce the same therapeutic effect when used appropriately.
- Undergo regulatory review for quality, safety, and efficacy.
- Are usually less expensive than brand-name drugs.

Inactive ingredients (such as fillers, binders, coloring agents, and preservatives) may differbutshouldnot significantlyaffecttherapeutic performance in most patients.

Characteristics of Brand-Name Drugs

Brand-name drugs:

- Are usually the first products introduced to the market. Require extensive research and development.
- Undergo comprehensive preclinical and clinical testing. Are protected by patents for a specified period.
- Are generally more expensive than generic equivalents.

Bioequivalence

Definition

Bioequivalence means that two pharmaceutical products have no clinically significant difference in the rate and extent of absorption when administered under similar conditions.

Regulatory agencies require generic drugs to demonstrate bioequivalence before approval.

Bioequivalence is commonly evaluated using:

- Maximum plasma concentration (Cmax)
- Time to maximum concentration (Tmax)
- Area under the plasma concentration-time curve (AUC)

Generic Substitution

Generic substitution is the practice of dispensing a generic drug instead of its brand-name equivalent.

Generic substitution is appropriate when:

- The products are therapeutically equivalent.
- Regulatory approval has been granted.
- National laws and institutional policies permit substitution.

Genericsubstitution canreducehealthcare costs while maintaining treatment effectiveness.

Therapeutic Equivalence

Twodrugs areconsidered therapeutically equivalent when they:

- Contain the same active ingredient.
- Have the same dosage form and strength.
- Demonstrate bioequivalence.
- Produce the same clinicaleffect andsafety profile when used as directed.

Advantages of Generic Drugs

Generic drugs provide numerous benefits.

Clinical Advantages

- Equivalent therapeutic efficacy.
- Comparable safety.
- Equivalent quality standards.
- Wide availability.

Economic Advantages

- Lower cost.
- Improved patient access to medications.
- Better medication adherence because of affordability.
- Reduced healthcare expenditure.

Advantages of Brand-Name Drugs

Brand-name drugs may offer certain advantages.

- Extensive clinical experience.
- Familiarity among healthcare professionals.
- Consistent product appearance.
- Availability of proprietary formulations or delivery systems.

Some brand-name products may include specialized formulations that are not immediatelyavailableasgeneric equivalents.

Potential Differences Between Generic and Brand-Name Drugs

Although therapeutically equivalent, generic and brand-name drugs may differ in:

- Tablet or capsule appearance
- Shape
- Color
- Inactive ingredients (excipients)
- Packaging
- Manufacturer

These differences usually do not affect clinical effectiveness.

Situations Where Brand-Name Prescribing May Be Preferred

Although generic drugs are appropriate for most patients, brand-name prescribing

may occasionally be considered for:

- Certain narrow therapeutic index (NTI) medications when clinically justified.
- Patients with documented allergy or intolerance to specific inactive ingredients.
- Modified-release or specialized drug delivery systems when no equivalent generic formulation is available.
- Clinical situations requiring strict product consistency, based on professional judgment and local guidelines.

Examples of drugs that may warrant careful consideration during product substitution include:

- Levothyroxine
- Tacrolimus
- Cyclosporine
- Certainantiepilepticmedications(depending on the clinical situation)

Role of Regulatory Agencies

National regulatory authorities evaluate generic drugs before approval.

They ensure that generic products meet standards for:

- Quality
- Safety
- Efficacy
- Manufacturing practices
- Bioequivalence

Examples of regulatory agencies include:

- U.S. Food and Drug Administration (FDA)
- European Medicines Agency (EMA)
- Medicines and Healthcare products Regulatory Agency (MHRA) (United Kingdom)

Clinical Importance

Healthcare professionals should:

- Prescribe using generic names whenever appropriate.
- Educate patients about generic substitution.
- Reassure patients regarding the effectiveness and safety of approved generic medications.
- Monitor therapeutic response after any medication change.
- Consider patient-specific factors before switching products in selected clinical situations.

Summary Table

Feature	Generic Drug	Brand-Name Drug
Active ingredient	Same	Original
Therapeutic effect	Equivalent	Original reference
Bioequivalence required	Yes	Not applicable
Cost	Usually lower	Usually higher
Patent protection	No	Yes (during patent period)
Marketing name	Generic (nonproprietary)	Trademark (proprietary)

Learning Objectives

After studying this chapter, you should be able to:

- Define generic and brand-name drugs.
- Differentiate between generic and brand-name medications.
- Explain the concepts of bioequivalence and therapeutic equivalence.
- Describe the advantages and limitations of generic substitution.
- Discuss the role of regulatory agencies in approving generic drugs.
- Apply principles of rational prescribing using generic medications.

Key Points to Remember

- Ageneric drug contains thesame active ingredient as the corresponding brand-name drug.
- Generic drugs must demonstrate bioequivalence before receiving regulatory approval.
- Approved generic drugs have comparable quality, safety, efficacy, dosage form, strength, and route of administration to their brand-name counterparts.
- Bioequivalence means there is no clinically significant difference in the rate and extent of drug absorption between the generic and brand-name products.
- Generic drugs are generally less expensive, improving patient access and medication adherence.
- Brand-name drugs are the original products developed and marketed under patent protection.
- Generic and brand-name drugs may differ in appearance, packaging, and inactive ingredients, but these differences usually do not affect therapeutic outcomes.
- Generic substitution is appropriate for most medications, although careful consideration may be needed for selected narrow therapeutic index drugs or specialized formulations.
- Prescribing by generic name promotes rational prescribing, reduces medication errors, and help slower healthcare costs.

Exam Pearls

- Generic (nonproprietary) name identifies the active ingredient, whereas the brand (trade) name is assigned by the manufacturer.
- Generic drugs must demonstrate bioequivalence to the reference brand-name product.
- Bioequivalence is evaluated using pharmacokinetic parameters such as Cmax, Tmax, and AUC.
- Approved generic drugs have the same active ingredient, strength, dosage form, route of administration, quality, safety, and therapeutic effect as the corresponding brand-name drug.
- Generic medications are generally more affordable because they do not require repeating the original drug development and clinical trials.
- Differences in color, shape, packaging, and inactive ingredients do not usually affect clinical efficacy.
- Levothyroxine, tacrolimus, cyclosporine, and certain antiepileptic drugs may require careful monitoring when switching between manufacturers because of their narrow therapeutic indices or product-specific considerations.
- Prescribingbygenericname isencouragedby mosthealthcaresystemsto improve medication safety, accessibility, and cost-effectiveness.

Rational Drug Use

Introduction

Rational Drug Use (RDU) is one of the fundamental principles of modern pharmacology and clinical medicine. It refers to the appropriate selection, prescribing, dispensing, and use of medicines to achieve the best possible
therapeutic outcomes while minimizing adverse effects, medication errors, antimicrobial resistance, and unnecessary healthcare costs.

The concept of rational drug use was introduced and promoted by the World Health Organization (WHO) to improve patient care and ensure the efficient use of healthcare resources. Irrational use of medicines remains a major global health problem and contributes to treatment failure, adverse drug reactions, drug resistance, and increased healthcare expenditures.

Healthcare professionals have a shared responsibility to promote the rational use of medicines through evidence-based prescribing, patient education, and continuous monitoring of treatment outcomes.

Definition

According to the World Health Organization (WHO):

"Rational use of medicines requires that patients receive medications appropriate to their clinical needs, in doses that meet their individual requirements, for an adequate periodof time, and at the lowest cost to themand their community."

Objectives of Rational Drug Use

- Thegoals ofrational drugusesareto:
- Maximize therapeutic effectiveness.
- Minimize adverse drug reactions.
- Prevent medication errors.
- Reduce unnecessary healthcare costs.
- Improve medication adherence.
- Prevent antimicrobial resistance.
- Promote patient safety.
- Optimize healthcare resources.

Principles of Rational Drug Use

Rational prescribing follows a systematic approach.

1. Accurate Diagnosis

Treatment should be based on a correct clinical diagnosis supported by:

- Medical history
- Physical examination
- Appropriate laboratory investigations
- Diagnostic imaging when indicated

2. Appropriate Drug Selection

Choose the most suitable medication based on:

- Proven efficacy
- Safety profile
- Patient characteristics
- Cost-effectiveness
- Availability
- Clinical guidelines

3. Individualized Drug Therapy

Drug therapy should be tailored according to:

- Age
- Body weight
- Pregnancy status
- Renal function
- Hepatic function
- Comorbidities
- Previous drug allergies
- Concurrent medications

4. Correct Dose

The prescribed dose should achieve therapeutic effectiveness while minimizing toxicity.

Dose adjustment may be necessary for:

- Children
- Older adults
- Patients with renal impairment
- Patients with hepaticimpairment

5. Appropriate Route of Administration

Select the safest and most effective route.

Examples include:

- Oral
- Intravenous
- Intramuscular
- Subcutaneous
- Topical
- Inhalational

6. Appropriate Duration of Therapy

Treatment should continue:

- Long enough to achieve cure or disease control.
- No longer than necessary to reduce adverse effects and resistance.

7. Patient Education

Patients should understand:

- Why the medicine is prescribed
- How to take it correctly
- Duration of treatment
- Possible adverse effects
- Drug interactions
- Storage instructions
- What to doifadoseismissed

8. Monitoring Therapy

Regular follow-up should assess:

- Therapeutic response
- Adverse drug reactions
- Medication adherence
- Laboratory investigations when indicated

The WHO Guide to Good Prescribing

The WHO recommends six steps for rational prescribing:

1. Define the patient's problem.
2. Specify the therapeutic objective.
3. Select the appropriate treatment.
4. Start the treatment with clear instructions.
5. Provide patient education and warnings.
6. Monitor treatment and discontinue therapy when appropriate.

Irrational Drug Use

Irrational drug use refers to the inappropriate use of medications that does not follow evidence-based principles.

Examples include:

- Polypharmacy without indication
- Unnecessary antibiotic prescribing
- Inappropriate use of injections
- Incorrect dosing
- Self-medication
- Overuse of vitamins and supplements without indication
- Failureto followtreatmentguidelines

Common Causes of Irrational Drug Use

Factors contributing to irrational prescribing include:

- Inadequate knowledge
- Diagnostic uncertainty
- Patient demand
- Pharmaceutical promotion
- Lack of clinical guidelines
- Poor communication
- Limited access to essential medicines
- Inadequate continuing medical education

Consequences of Irrational Drug Use

Irrational medication use may lead to:

- Treatment failure
- Adverse drug reactions
- Drug toxicity
- Antimicrobial resistance
- Increased healthcare costs
- Medication errors
- Poor patient adherence
- Increased hospitalization
- Reduced qualityoflife

Polypharmacy

Polypharmacy is commonly defined as the use of five or more medications simultaneously.

Although sometimes clinically appropriate, unnecessary polypharmacy increases the risk of:

- Drug interactions
- Adverse drug reactions
- Medication errors
- Poor adherence
- Hospitalization

Healthcare professionals should regularly review medication lists to discontinue unnecessary drugs.

Antimicrobial Stewardship

Antimicrobial stewardship is an important component of rational drug use.

Its goals include:

- Appropriate antibiotic selection
- Correct dose
- Correct duration
- Prevention of antimicrobial resistance
- Reduction of unnecessary antibiotic use

Examples of good stewardship include:

- Prescribing antibiotics only for confirmed or strongly suspected bacterial infections.
- Using culture and sensitivity results whenever possible.
- Avoidingantibioticsforviral illnessessuch as the common cold.

Role of Essential Medicines

The use of essential medicines supports rational drug use by ensuring that patients

receive medications that are:

- Effective
- Safe
- Affordable
- Evidence-based
- Readily available

Role of Healthcare Professionals

Physicians

- Establish accurate diagnoses.
- Prescribe evidence-based therapy.
- Review medication interactions.
- Monitor treatment effectiveness.

Pharmacists

- Verify prescriptions.
- Counsel patients.
- Detect medication errors.
- Monitor for drug interactions.

Nurses

- Administer medications safely.
- Monitor patient response.
- Educate patients.
- Report adverse drug reactions.

Patients

- Follow prescribed instructions.
- Report adverse effects.
- Avoid sharing medications.
- Complete prescribed treatment courses.

Strategies to Promote Rational Drug Use

Effective strategies include:

- Evidence-based clinical guidelines
- Continuing professional education
- Standard treatment protocols
- Essential Medicines Lists
- Electronic prescribing systems
- Medication reconciliation
- Drug utilization reviews
- Antimicrobial stewardship programs
- Patient education
- Pharmacovigilance

Clinical Importance

Rational drug use:

- Improves therapeutic outcomes.
- Enhances patient safety.
- Reduces adverse drug reactions.
- Prevents medication errors.
- Slows the development of antimicrobial resistance.
- Improves medication adherence.
- Optimizes healthcare resources.
- Reduces healthcare costs.

Summary Table

Principle	**Purpose**
Accurate diagnosis	Appropriate treatment selection
Appropriate drug	Maximum efficacy with minimum harm
Individualized therapy	Patient-specific treatment
Correct dose	Maximize efficacy and reduce toxicity
Appropriate duration	Prevent treatment failure and resistance
Patient education	Improve adherence and safety
Monitoring	Detect efficacy and adverse effects

Learning Objectives

Afterstudyingthis chapter,youshould be able to:

- Define rational drug use.
- Explain the WHO definition of rational medicine use.
- Describe the principles of rational prescribing.
- Identify causes and consequences of irrational drug use.
- Discuss the importance of antimicrobial stewardship and essential medicines.
- Apply rational drug use principles in everyday clinical practice.

Key Points to Remember

- Rational DrugUse (RDU) means prescribing medications that are appropriate for the patient's clinical needs, in the correct dose, for the appropriate duration, and at the lowest reasonable cost.
- Rational prescribing begins with an accurate diagnosis and evidence-based drug selection.
- Drug therapy should always be individualized, taking into account age, body weight, renal and hepatic function, pregnancy, allergies, comorbidities, and concurrent medications.
- Patient education and regular monitoring are essential to ensure treatment effectiveness, medication adherence, and early detection of adverse drug reactions.
- Polypharmacy increases the risk of drug interactions, adverse drug reactions, medication errors, and poor adherence, particularly in older adults.
- Antimicrobial stewardship promotes the appropriate use of antibiotics and helps reduce antimicrobial resistance.
- The use of Essential Medicines supports rational prescribing by promoting access to safe, effective, quality-assured, and affordable medications.
- Rational drug use improves patient safety, therapeutic outcomes, and the efficient use of healthcare resources.

Exam Pearls

- WHO Definition: Patients should receive medicines appropriate to their clinical needs, in doses that meet their individual requirements, for an adequate duration, and at the lowest cost to both the patient and the community.
- The key elements of rational prescribing are the right patient, the right drug, the right dose, the right route, the right duration, and appropriate monitoring.
- An accurate diagnosis is the foundation of rational drug therapy.
- Polypharmacy is commonly defined as the use of five or more medications and is associated with increased risks of adverse drug reactions and drug interactions.
- Antibiotics should not be prescribed for viral infections such as the common cold or uncomplicated influenza.
- Antimicrobial stewardship aims to optimize antibiotic therapy while reducing antimicrobial resistance.
- Essential Medicines Lists (EMLs) promote equitable access to effective, safe, and cost-effective medications.
- Regular medication review, patient counseling, medication reconciliation, and pharmacovigilance are key strategies for promoting rational drug use.
- Rational drug use is a shared responsibility of physicians, pharmacists, nurses, and patients.

Principles of Evidence-Based Pharmacotherapy

Introduction

Evidence-Based Pharmacotherapy (EBP) is the application of the best available scientific evidence, combined with clinical expertise and patient preferences, to select the safest and most effective drug therapy for individual patients. It is a cornerstone of modern clinical practice and promotes rational prescribing, improved therapeutic outcomes, and patient safety.

The rapid expansion of medical research has resulted in an enormous amount of information about medications. Healthcare professionals must be able to critically evaluate this evidence and apply it appropriately in clinical decision-making.

Evidence-based pharmacotherapy helps clinicians choose treatments that are supported by high-quality research rather than tradition, anecdotal experience, or personal preference.

Definition

Evidence-Based Pharmacotherapy is the process of making drug therapy decisions by integrating:

- The best available scientific evidence.
- Clinical expertise.
- Patient values and preferences.

These three components work together to provide individualized, safe, and effective patient care.

Components of Evidence-Based Pharmacotherapy

Evidence-based pharmacotherapy is built upon three essential pillars.

1. Best Available Scientific Evidence

Drug therapy should be based on reliable and up-to-date scientific research, including:

- Randomized controlled trials (RCTs)
- Systematic reviews
- Meta-analyses
- Clinical practice guidelines
- High-quality observational studies (when appropriate)

2. Clinical Expertise

Healthcare professionals use their knowledge and experience to:

- Interpret scientific evidence.
- Assess disease severity.
- Recognize contraindications.
- Identify potential adverse effects.
- Individualize treatment.
- Monitor therapeutic response.

3. Patient Values and Preferences

Treatment decisions should consider:

- Patient preferences
- Cultural beliefs
- Lifestyle
- Financial considerations
- Treatment goals
- Ability to adhere to therapy
- Shared decision-making improves patient satisfaction and medication adherence.

Steps in Evidence-Based Pharmacotherapy

The evidence-based approach follows a systematic process.

Step 1: Formulate a Clinical Question

Clinical questions should be focused and answerable.

The PICO format is commonly used.

Component	Description
P	Patient or Problem
I	Intervention
C	Comparison
O	Outcome

Example

In adults with hypertension (P), does an ACE inhibitor (I), compared with a beta blocker (C), reduce cardiovascular mortality (O)?

Step 2: Search for Evidence

Reliable sources include:

- Clinical practice guidelines
- Systematic reviews
- Medical databases
- Peer-reviewed journals
- Drug formularies
- National and international treatment guidelines

Step 3: Critically Appraise the Evidence

Evaluate:

- Study design
- Methodological quality
- Risk of bias
- Statistical significance
- Clinical relevance
- Applicability to the patient

Step 4: Apply the Evidence

Consider:

- Individual patient characteristics
- Benefits versus risks
- Contraindications
- Drug interactions
- Cost
- Patient preferences

Step 5: Evaluate Outcomes

Monitor:

- Therapeutic response
- Adverse drug reactions
- Laboratory values
- Medication adherence
- Patient satisfaction

Modify therapy when necessary.

Hierarchy of Evidence

Not allscientific evidence hasequal strength.

The hierarchy of evidence ranks study designs according to their reliability.

Level	Type of Evidence
1	Systematic reviews and meta-analyses
2	Randomized controlled trials (RCTs)
3	Cohort studies
4	Case-control studies
5	Case series and case reports
6	Expert opinion and laboratory research

Higher levels generally providestrongerevidencefor therapeutic decisions.

Clinical Practice Guidelines

Clinical practice guidelinesaresystematically developed recommendations based on current scientific evidence.

They help clinicians:

- Select appropriate medications.
- Standardize treatment.
- Improve patient outcomes.
- Reduce unnecessary variation in care.

Examples include guidelines for:

- Hypertension
- Diabetes mellitus
- Heart failure
- Asthma
- Chronic kidney disease

Benefits of Evidence-Based Pharmacotherapy

Evidence-based pharmacotherapy:

- Improves therapeutic outcomes.
- Enhances patient safety.
- Reduces adverse drug reactions.
- Supports rational prescribing.
- Promotes cost-effective therapy.
- Improves medication adherence.
- Reduces unnecessary drug use.
- Supports continuous professionaldevelopment.

Limitations of Evidence-Based Pharmacotherapy

Despite its advantages, challenges include:

- Limited evidence for rare diseases.
- Underrepresentation of certain patient populations in clinical trials.
- Conflicting study results.
- Rapidly evolving medical knowledge.
- Limited access to high-quality evidence in some settings.
- Variability in patient preferences and clinical circumstances.

Clinicaljudgmentremainsessential when applying evidence to individual patients.

Shared Decision-Making

Evidence-based pharmacotherapy encourages collaboration between healthcare professionals and patients.

Shared decision-making includes:

- Explaining treatment options.
- Discussing benefits and risks.
- Considering patient preferences.
- Respecting patient autonomy.
- Agreeing on a treatment plan together.

Role of Pharmacovigilance

Evidencecontinues toaccumulateaftermedications are marketed.

Pharmacovigilance helps identify:

- Rare adverse drug reactions.
- Long-term safety concerns.
- Drug interactions.
- Medication errors.
- New safety warnings.

Thisongoingprocesscontributes to safer prescribing and updates clinical guidelines.

Clinical Importance

Evidence-based pharmacotherapy enables clinicians to:

- Prescribe the most effective medications.
- Minimize unnecessary treatments.
- Improve patient safety.
- Optimize healthcare resources.
- Individualize drug therapy.
- Promote high-quality patient care.

Summary Table

Principle	Purpose
Best availableevidence	Supports effective treatment decisions
Clinical expertise	Individualizes therapy
Patient preferences	Promotes shared decision-making
Critical appraisal	Ensures evidence quality
Outcome evaluation	Measures treatment success

Learning Objectives

After studying this chapter, you should be able to:

- Define evidence-based pharmacotherapy.
- Describe the three pillars of evidence-based pharmacotherapy.
- Explain the steps involved in evidence-based clinical decision-making.
- Describe the hierarchy of scientific evidence.
- Discuss the importance of clinical practice guidelines.
- Apply evidence-based principles to rational prescribing.

Key Points to Remember

- Evidence-Based Pharmacotherapy(EBP) integrates the best available scientific evidence, clinical expertise, and patient values to optimize medication therapy.
- Treatment decisions should be based on high-quality scientific evidence whenever available.
- The PICO framework helps formulate focused clinical questions.
- Evidence should be critically appraised for validity, reliability, clinical relevance, and applicability before being applied to patient care.
- Systematic reviews and meta-analyses provide the highest level of evidence for most therapeutic interventions, followed by randomized controlled trials (RCTs).
- Clinical practice guidelines translate scientific evidence into practical recommendations for patient care.
- Shared decision-making improves medication adherence, patient satisfaction, and therapeutic outcomes.
- Continuous monitoring and pharmacovigilance are essential because new evidence may change recommendations over time.
- Evidence-based pharmacotherapy promotes safe, effective, patient-centered, and cost-effective prescribing.

Exam Pearls

- Evidence-Based Pharmacotherapy combines scientific evidence, clinical expertise, and patient preferences.
- The PICO model stands for Patient (or Problem), Intervention, Comparison, and Outcome.
- Systematic reviews and meta-analyses generally provide the highest level of clinical evidence for treatment decisions.
- Randomized controlled trials (RCTs) are considered the gold standard for evaluating the efficacy of therapeutic interventions.
- Clinical decisions should consider benefits, risks, contraindications, drug interactions, patient preferences, and cost-effectiveness.
- Clinical practice guidelines are evidence-based recommendations designed to improve consistency and quality of patient care.
- Shared decision-making strengthens the partnership between healthcare professionals and patients and supports adherence to treatment.
- Evidence-based pharmacotherapy requires continuous evaluation, as new research and pharmacovigilance data may modify existing recommendations.
- High-quality evidence should guide—but not replace—clinical judgment, which remains essential for individualized patient care.

Part I – General Principles of Pharmacology

Multiple Choice Questions (MCQs)

Instructions

- Choose the single best answer (SBA) for each question.
- Each question has one correct answer.
- Read all options carefully before selecting your answer.
- An answer key with detailed explanations is provided at the end of this section.

Examination Blueprint

Topic	No. of MCQs
Definition and Scope of Pharmacology	5
Branches of Pharmacology	5
Drug Classification	5
Sources of Drugs	5
Routes of DrugAdministration	8
Drug Receptors	8
Mechanisms ofDrugAction	8
Agonists and Antagonists	8
Dose–Response Relationships	8
Potency and Efficacy	6
Therapeutic Index	6
Drug Selectivity	5
Adverse DrugReactions	8
Drug Safety	4
Medication Errors	4
Essential Medicines	3
Generic and Brand-Name Drugs	3
Rational Drug Use	3
Principles of Evidence-Based Pharmacotherapy	2
Total	100 MCQs

Types of Questions Included

The MCQ section includes a balanced mix of:

- Recall (Knowledge)
- Understanding (Concepts)
- Clinical application
- Drug calculations
- Case-based questions
- Clinical reasoning
- Patient safety
- Pharmacovigilance
- Rational prescribing
- Evidence-based medicine

Difficulty Distribution

Difficulty Level	Percentage	Number of Questions
Easy	30%	30
Moderate	50%	50
Difficult	20%	20

Question Format

Each question contains:

- One clinical or factual stem
- Four answer options (A–D)
- One best answer
- Detailed explanation
- Learning point
- Reference to the relevant chapter

Clinical Emphasis

Approximately40–50%ofthe MCQs are case-based to reflect modern medical licensing and nursing examinations.

Clinical scenarios assess the learner's ability to apply pharmacological principles in real-worldpatient carerather thansimply recalling facts.

Educational Objectives

UponcompletingthisMCQ section,readers should be able to:

- Apply the fundamental principles of pharmacology in clinical practice.
- Select the most appropriate medication based on efficacy, safety, and patient-specific factors.
- Interpret dose–response relationships and therapeutic indices.
- Recognize adverse drug reactions and medication errors.
- Practice rational prescribing and evidence-based pharmacotherapy.
- Improve readiness for undergraduate, postgraduate, and professional licensing examinations.

Suggested Examination Time

- 100 MCQs
- 120 minutes
- Approximately 1.2 minutes per question

Scoring Guide

Score	Performance
90–100%	Excellent – Examination Ready
80–89%	Very Good – Minor Revision Needed
70–79%	Good – Continue Practice
60–69%	Fair – Requires Further Study
Below 60%	Significant Revision Recommended

Recommended Audience

This MCQ section is suitable for:

- Medical students
- Nursing students
- Pharmacy students
- Physician Assistant students
- Clinical Pharmacology trainees
- Medical interns
- Residents
- General practitioners
- Nurses preparing for licensing examinations
- Healthcare professionals seeking to refresh their pharmacology knowledge

Part I – General Principles of Pharmacology

MCQs 1–20

MCQ 1

Pharmacology is best defined as the science that studies:

A. Human anatomy only

B. Drugs and their interactions with living organisms

C. Microorganisms causing disease

D. Surgical treatment of diseases

Answer: B

Explanation: Pharmacology is the scientific study of drugs, including their sources, properties, mechanisms of action, therapeutic uses, adverse effects, and interactions with living organisms.

Clinical Pearl: Pharmacology forms the scientific basis for rational prescribing and safe medication use.

MCQ 2

Which branch of pharmacology studies the effects of drugs on the body?

A. Pharmacokinetics

B. Pharmacodynamics

C. Toxicology

D. Pharmacogenomics

Answer: B

Explanation: Pharmacodynamics describes what the drug does to the body, including receptor interactions and physiological effects.

Clinical Pearl: Pharmacodynamics explains drug efficacy, potency, and receptor activity.

MCQ 3

Pharmacokinetics primarily describes:

A. Drug toxicity

B. Drug interactions

C. What the body does to the drug

D. Drug allergy

Answer: C

Explanation: Pharmacokinetics includes drug Absorption, Distribution, Metabolism, and Excretion (ADME).

Clinical Pearl: Remember the acronym ADME.

MCQ 4

Which process is NOT part of pharmacokinetics?

A. Absorption

B. Distribution

C. Receptor binding

D. Elimination

Answer: C

Explanation: Receptor binding is a pharmacodynamic process.

Clinical Pearl: Pharmacokinetics follows the journey of the drug through the body.

MCQ 5

The official nonproprietary name of a drug is called its:

A. Brand name

B. Chemical name

C. Generic name

D. Trade name

Answer: C

Explanation: The generic name is the internationally recognized nonproprietary name of the active ingredient.

Clinical Pearl: Prescribing by generic name reduces medication errors and healthcare costs.

MCQ 6

Which of the following is a brand (trade) name?

A. Ibuprofen

B. Amoxicillin

C. Advil®

D. Metformin

Answer: C

Explanation: Advil® is a brand name for ibuprofen.

Clinical Pearl: One generic drug may have multiple brand names.

MCQ 7

Drugs derived from microorganisms include:

A. Digoxin

B. Penicillin

C. Insulin

D. Atropine

Answer: B

Explanation: Penicillin is produced by the fungus Penicillium.

Clinical Pearl: Many antibiotics originate from microorganisms.

MCQ 8

Which route of administration provides the fastest onset of action?

A. Oral

B. Intramuscular

C. Intravenous

D. Subcutaneous

Answer: C

Explanation: Intravenous administration delivers the drug directly into the bloodstream, producing an immediate effect.

Clinical Pearl: IV administration has 100% bioavailability.

MCQ 9

The oral route of drug administration is characterized by:

A. Complete avoidance of first-pass metabolism

B. Immediate drug effect

C. Possible first-pass hepatic metabolism

D. Highest bioavailability

Answer: C

Explanation: Drugs administered orally may undergo first-pass metabolism in the liver before reaching systemic circulation.

Clinical Pearl: First-pass metabolism may reduce drug bioavailability.

MCQ 10

The transdermal route is most suitable for drugs requiring:

A. Immediate emergency treatment

B. Sustained systemic delivery

C. Rapid anesthesia

D. Intravenous access

Answer: B

Explanation: Transdermal patches provide slow, continuous drug absorption over an extended period.

Clinical Pearl: Examples include nicotine and fentanyl patches.

MCQ 11

Drug receptors are usually:

A. Plasma proteins

B. Enzymes

C. Macromolecules that bind drugs and initiate a response

D. Red blood cells

Answer: C

Explanation: Most drug receptors are proteins located on cell membranes or inside cells.

Clinical Pearl: Drug-receptor interaction is the basis of pharmacodynamics.

MCQ 12

An agonist is a drug that:

A. Blocks receptor activation

B. Binds to a receptor and activates it

C. Destroys receptors

D. Prevents drug metabolism

Answer: B

Explanation: Agonists possess both receptor affinity and intrinsic activity.

Clinical Pearl: Full agonists produce the maximum biological response.

MCQ 13

A competitive antagonist:

A. Irreversibly destroys receptors

B. Binds reversibly to the receptor without activating it

C. Produces maximal receptor activation

D. Enhances agonist activity

Answer: B

Explanation: Competitive antagonists compete with agonists for the same receptor and their effects can often be overcome by increasing agonist concentration.

Clinical Pearl: Naloxone is a competitive opioid receptor antagonist.

MCQ 14

The relationship between drug dose and response is described by the:

A. Therapeutic index

B. Dose–response curve

C. Half-life

D. Volume of distribution

Answer: B

Explanation: The dose–response curve illustrates how increasing drug doses affect the magnitude of the response.

Clinical Pearl: Dose–response curves help compare drug potency and efficacy.

MCQ 15

A drug requiring a smaller dose to produce the same effect is considered more:

A. Toxic

B. Selective

C. Potent

D. Effective

Answer: C

Explanation: Potency refers to the amount of drug needed to produce a given effect.

Clinical Pearl: Potency does not necessarily indicate greater clinical benefit.

MCQ 16

The maximum effect a drug can produce is called its:

A. Potency

B. Efficacy

C. Bioavailability

D. Clearance

Answer: B

Explanation: Efficacy (Emax) is the greatest therapeutic response achievable with a drug.

Clinical Pearl: Efficacy is generally more clinically important than potency.

MCQ 17

A drug with a high therapeutic index is generally considered:

A. Less effective

B. More toxic

C. Safer

D. Less potent

Answer: C

Explanation: A high therapeutic index indicates a wide margin between effective and toxic doses.

Clinical Pearl: Penicillins generally have a wider therapeutic index than digoxin.

MCQ 18

Drug selectivity refers to a drug's ability to:

A. Act only on one organ

B. Preferentially act on one receptor or target over others

C. Eliminate rapidly

D. Avoid metabolism

Answer: B

Explanation: Selective drugs preferentially bind certain receptors but may affect others at higher doses.

Clinical Pearl: No drug is completely specific.

MCQ 19

A patient develops severe anaphylaxis immediately after receiving penicillin. This is an example of which type of adverse drug reaction?

A. Type A (Augmented)

B. Type B (Bizarre)

C. Type C (Chronic)

D. Type E (Withdrawal)

Answer: B

Explanation: Penicillin-induced anaphylaxis is an unpredictable, immune-mediated Type B adverse drug reaction.

Clinical Pearl: Type B reactions are uncommon but may be life-threatening.

MCQ 20

Which statement best describes rational drug use?

A. Prescribing the newest medication available

B. Prescribing multiple drugs for every disease

C. Using medications appropriate to the patient's clinical needs, in the correct dose and duration, at the lowest appropriate cost

D. Prescribing antibiotics for all febrile illnesses

Answer: C

Explanation: According to the World Health Organization, rational drug use means providing the right medicine, at the right dose, for the right duration, and at the lowest cost to the patient and the community.

Clinical Pearl: Rational prescribing improves therapeutic outcomes, reduces adverse drug reactions, and helps prevent antimicrobial resistance.

Part I – General Principles of Pharmacology

MCQs 21–40

MCQ 21

Which statement best describes bioavailability?

A. The rate of drug metabolism

B. The fraction of an administered dose that reaches the systemic circulation unchanged C. The duration of drug action

D. The degree of protein binding

Answer: B

Explanation: Bioavailability refers to the proportion of an administered drug that reaches the systemic circulation in an active form. Intravenous drugs have 100% bioavailability.

Clinical Pearl: Oral drugs usually have lower bioavailability because of incomplete absorption and first-pass metabolism.

MCQ 22

Which route of administration completely avoids first-pass hepatic metabolism?

A. Oral

B. Rectal

C. Intravenous

D. Sublingual

Answer: C

Explanation: Intravenous administration delivers the drug directly into the bloodstream, bypassing the liver during initial circulation.

Clinical Pearl: Sublingual drugs also largely avoidfirst-pass metabolism.

MCQ 23

A patient with severe vomiting requires immediate medication. Which route is most appropriate?

A. Oral

B. Intravenous

C. Topical

D. Rectal

Answer: B

Explanation: Intravenous administration provides rapid drug delivery and is preferred when oral administration is not possible.

Clinical Pearl: IV therapy is commonly used in emergency situations.

MCQ 24

Which receptor type is directly coupled to ion channels?

A. G protein-coupled receptor

B. Enzyme-linked receptor

C. Ligand-gated ion channel

D. Intracellular receptor

Answer: C

Explanation: Ligand-gated ion channels open or close in response to ligand binding, producing rapid cellular responses.

Clinical Pearl: Nicotinic acetylcholine receptors are classic ligand-gated ion channels.

MCQ 25

Intracellular receptors are primarily activated by:

A. Large protein molecules

B. Peptide hormones

C. Lipid-soluble drugs

D. Neurotransmitters

Answer: C

Explanation: Lipid-soluble drugs can cross the cell membrane and bind intracellular receptors.

Clinical Pearl: Steroid hormones act through intracellular receptors.

MCQ 26

A partial agonist produces:

A. No receptor activation

B. Maximum receptor activation

C. Less than the maximum response even when all receptors are occupied

D. Irreversible receptor blockade

Answer: C

Explanation: Partial agonists have affinity for receptors but lower intrinsic activity than full agonists.

Clinical Pearl: Buprenorphine is an example of a partial opioid agonist.

MCQ 27

Which pharmacodynamic parameter represents the maximum achievable drug effect?

A. ED50

B. Half-life

C. Emax

D. Clearance

Answer: C

Explanation: Emax represents the maximum efficacy that a drug can produce.

Clinical Pearl: Increasing the dose beyond Emax does not increase the therapeutic response.

MCQ 28

The ED50 of a drug refers to the dose that:

A. Produces toxicity in 50% of patients

B. Produces the desired effect in 50% of individuals

C. Is lethal in 50% of animals

D. Is eliminated in 50% of patients

Answer: B

Explanation: ED50 (Median Effective Dose) is the dose producing the desired therapeutic effect in 50% of the population.

Clinical Pearl: ED50 is commonly used to compare drug potency.

MCQ 29

Which drug characteristic is reflected by the position of the dose–response curve along the x-axis?

A. Toxicity

B. Efficacy

C. Potency

D. Selectivity

Answer: C

Explanation: A leftward shift indicates greater potency because less drug is required to achieve the same effect.

Clinical Pearl: Potency is determined by dose, not by maximal effect.

MCQ 30

Two drugs produce the same maximum effect, but Drug A requires a lower dose than Drug B. Drug A is:

A. More effective

B. More potent

C. More selective

D. Less safe

Answer: B

Explanation: Drug A is more potent because it achieves the same effect at a lower dose.

Clinical Pearl: Greater potency does not necessarily mean better clinical efficacy.

MCQ 31

Which drug is well known for having a narrow therapeutic index?

A. Amoxicillin

B. Digoxin

C. Paracetamol (Acetaminophen)

D. Cetirizine

Answer: B

Explanation: Digoxin has a narrow therapeutic index, requiring careful dose adjustment and monitoring.

Clinical Pearl: Drugs with narrow therapeutic indices often require therapeutic drug monitoring.

MCQ 32

Which patient is at the greatest risk of developing adverse drug reactions?

A. Healthy young adult

B. Middle-aged athlete

C. Older adult taking multiple medications

D. Healthy teenager

Answer: C

Explanation: Older adults with polypharmacy have increased susceptibility to adverse drug reactions.

Clinical Pearl: Renal impairment and multiple comorbidities further increase the risk.

MCQ 33

Warfarin-induced bleeding is an example of which type of adverse drug reaction?

A. Type A

B. Type B

C. Type D

D. Type E

Answer: A

Explanation: Bleeding from warfarin is predictable, dose dependent, and therefore classified as a Type A ADR.

Clinical Pearl: Type A reactions account for most adverse drug reactions.

MCQ 34

Abrupt discontinuation of long-term corticosteroid therapy may result in:

A. Type A reaction

B. Type B reaction

C. Type E reaction

D. Type F reaction

Answer: C

Explanation: Withdrawal of corticosteroids may cause adrenal insufficiency, a classic Type E reaction.

Clinical Pearl: Corticosteroids should usually be tapered gradually.

MCQ 35

Which of the following best describes pharmacovigilance?

A. Drug manufacturing

B. Monitoring drug prices

C. Detection, assessment, and prevention of adverse drug reactions

D. Drug marketing

Answer: C

Explanation: Pharmacovigilance focuses on identifying and preventing medication-related harm after drugs enter clinical use.

Clinical Pearl: Healthcare professionals should report serious and unexpected adverse drug reactions.

MCQ 36

Which is considered a high-alert medication?

A. Vitamin C

B. Warfarin

C. Calcium carbonate

D. Loratadine

Answer: B

Explanation: Warfarin has a high risk of causing serious harm if used incorrectly.

Clinical Pearl: Other high-alert medications include insulin, heparin, opioids, and chemotherapy agents.

MCQ 37

Medication reconciliation is primarily intended to prevent:

A. Drug manufacturing errors

B. Drug omissions, duplications, and interactions

C. Drug allergies

D. Drug dependence

Answer: B

Explanation: Medication reconciliation compares current medications with new prescriptions during transitions of care.

Clinical Pearl: It should be performed at admission, transfer, and discharge.

MCQ 38

According to the WHO, essential medicines should be:

A. Available only in tertiary hospitals

B. Expensive and highly specialized

C. Available at all times in adequate quantities and affordable

D. Restricted to emergency departments

Answer: C

Explanation: Essential medicines should be continuously available, affordable, and of assured quality.

Clinical Pearl: The WHO Model List of Essential Medicines guides national medicine policies.

MCQ 39

An approved generic drug must have the same:

A. Tablet color only

B. Packaging only

C. Active ingredient, dosage form, strength, and therapeutic effect as the brand-name drug

D. Manufacturer

Answer: C

Explanation: Generic drugs must demonstrate bioequivalence and therapeutic equivalence to the reference product.

Clinical Pearl: Generic substitution improves access to affordable medications.

MCQ 40

Which of the following is the best example of evidence-based pharmacotherapy?

A. Prescribing a drug because a colleague recommends it

B. Choosing therapy based solely on patient preference

C. Selecting medication using current clinical evidence, professional judgment, and patient preferences

D. Always prescribing the newest available medication

Answer: C

Explanation: Evidence-based pharmacotherapy integrates the best available research evidence with clinical expertise and patient values to achieve optimal therapeutic outcomes.

Clinical Pearl: Evidence-based prescribing improves patient safety, treatment effectiveness, and cost-effectiveness.

MCQ 41

A patient receives nitroglycerin sublingually for acute angina. The main advantage of the sublingual route is that it:

A. Produces sustained drug release for several days

B. Avoids first-pass hepatic metabolism and provides rapid absorption

C. Is less expensive than oral administration

D. Prevents all adverse drug reactions

Answer: B

Explanation: Sublingual administration allows rapid absorption through the oral mucosa directly into the systemic circulation, largely bypassing first-pass hepatic metabolism.

Clinical Pearl: Sublingual nitroglycerin typically begins to relieve angina within minutes.

MCQ 42

Which of the following is an example of a pharmacodynamic process?

A. Drug metabolism by the liver

B. Drug excretion by the kidneys

C. Binding of a drug to its receptor

D. Drug absorption from the intestine

Answer: C

Explanation: Pharmacodynamics describes the interaction between drugs and their receptors and the resulting biological effects.

Clinical Pearl: Pharmacodynamics answers the question: What does the drug do to the body?

MCQ 43

Which statement regarding receptor affinity is correct?

A. It describes the maximum effect produced by a drug.

B. It refers to the ability of a drug to bind to its receptor.

C. It measures drug elimination.

D. It determines drug bioavailability.

Answer: B

Explanation: Affinity is the tendency of a drug to bind to its receptor. High-affinity drugs bind more readily.

Clinical Pearl: Affinity and intrinsic activity together determine the pharmacological response.

MCQ 44

Which receptor type commonly activates second messengers such as cyclic AMP (cAMP)?

A. Ligand-gated ion channels

B. G protein-coupled receptors (GPCRs)

C. Intracellular receptors

D. Voltage-gated ion channels

Answer: B

Explanation: GPCRs activate intracellular signaling pathways involving second messengers such as cAMP and IP_3.

Clinical Pearl: GPCRs are the targets of a large proportion of clinically used medications.

MCQ 45

A noncompetitive antagonist differs from a competitive antagonist because it:

A. Increases receptor activation

B. Cannot be overcome by increasing the agonist concentration

C. Has greater potency

D. Produces maximal receptor activation

Answer: B

Explanation: Noncompetitive antagonists reduce the maximum response and cannot usually be overcome by increasing agonist concentration.

Clinical Pearl: Noncompetitive antagonists decrease drug efficacy rather than simply shifting the dose-response curve.

MCQ 46

Increasing the dose of a full agonist beyond its maximal efficacy (Emax) will:

A. Increase the maximum response further

B. Decrease potency

C. Produce no additional therapeutic effect but may increase toxicity

D. Convert it into a partial agonist

Answer: C

Explanation: Once Emax is reached, higher doses do not improve efficacy but increase the risk of adverse effects.

Clinical Pearl: "More drug" does not always mean "more benefit."

MCQ 47

Which factor is most likely to reduce the therapeutic index of a drug?

A. Wide margin between effective and toxic doses

B. Narrow difference between effective and toxic doses

C. High bioavailability

D. High receptor selectivity

Answer: B

Explanation: A narrow therapeutic index indicates that toxic effects occur at doses close to therapeutic doses.

Clinical Pearl: Digoxin, lithium, and warfarin require careful monitoring because of their narrow therapeutic indices.

MCQ 48

Drug selectivity is best described as the ability of a drug to:

A. Produce no adverse effects

B. Bind preferentially to a particular receptor or tissue

C. Eliminate rapidly from the body

D. Cross the blood-brain barrier

Answer: B

Explanation: Selective drugs preferentially interact with specific receptors, although complete specificity is rare.

Clinical Pearl: Selectivity often decreases as drug doses increase.

MCQ 49

Which adverse drug reaction is most likely to occur after prolonged drug therapy? A.

Type A

B. Type B

C. Type C

D. Type F

Answer: C

Explanation: Type C (Chronic) reactions are associated with long-term drug use and cumulative exposure.

Clinical Pearl: Long-term corticosteroid therapy causing osteoporosis is a classic example.

MCQ 50

Failure of an oral contraceptive due to rifampicin-induced enzyme induction is classified as:

A. Type A ADR

B. Type B ADR

C. Type E ADR

D. Type F ADR

Answer: D

Explanation: Type F reactions represent failure of therapy, often caused by drug interactions or inadequate dosing.

Clinical Pearl: Rifampicin induces hepatic enzymes and reduces the effectiveness of many medications.

MCQ 51

Which patient characteristic most commonly requires dose adjustment?

A. Brown eye color

B. Renal impairment

C. Left-handedness

D. Blood group O

Answer: B

Explanation: Many drugs are eliminated by the kidneys; impaired renal function can lead to drug accumulation and toxicity.

Clinical Pearl: Always assess kidney function before prescribing renally eliminated drugs.

MCQ 52

Which of the following is an important strategy for preventing medication errors?

A. Using abbreviations whenever possible

B. Confirming patient identity before medication administration

C. Prescribing multiple drugs without review

D. Ignoring patient allergies if the reaction occurred years earlier

Answer: B

Explanation: Correct patient identification is one of the fundamental principles of medication safety.

Clinical Pearl: Always verify at least two patient identifiers before administering medication.

MCQ 53

Which organization introduced the concept of Essential Medicines?

A. American Medical Association (AMA)

B. World Health Organization (WHO)

C. Centers for Disease Control and Prevention (CDC)

D. International Committee of the Red Cross (ICRC)

Answer: B

Explanation: The WHO introduced the Essential Medicines concept in 1977 to improve access to effective, safe, and affordable medicines.

Clinical Pearl: The WHO Model List serves as a guide for national essential medicines lists.

MCQ 54

Which statement regarding generic drugs is TRUE?

A. They contain different active ingredients than brand-name drugs.

B. They must demonstrate bioequivalence to the reference product.

C. They are less effective than brand-name drugs.

D. They are approved without regulatory review.

Answer: B

Explanation: Approved generic drugs must demonstrate bioequivalence and meet the same quality, safety, and efficacy standards as the reference product.

Clinical Pearl: Generic substitution is appropriate for most medications.

MCQ 55

Which of the following best reflects rational drug prescribing?

A. Prescribing antibiotics for every patient with fever

B. Choosing medications supported by evidence and tailored to the patient's needs

C. Prescribing the most expensive medication available

D. Prescribing medications requested by the patient without assessment

Answer: B

Explanation: Rational prescribing requires selecting evidence-based therapy appropriate for the patient's diagnosis and clinical condition.

Clinical Pearl: Rational prescribing improves outcomes while reducing unnecessary costs.

MCQ 56

The PICO model is primarily used to:

A. Classify adverse drug reactions

B. Formulate answerable clinical questions

C. Measure drug potency

D. Calculate drug half-life

Answer: B

Explanation: PICO stands for Patient (or Problem), Intervention, Comparison, and Outcome.

Clinical Pearl: PICO is widely used in evidence-based medicine to guide literature searches.

MCQ 57

Which type of scientific evidence generally provides the highest level of evidence for therapeutic interventions?

A. Expert opinion

B. Case reports

C. Randomized controlled trials

D. Systematic reviews and meta-analyses

Answer: D

Explanation: Systematic reviews and meta-analyses synthesize results from multiple high-quality studies and generally provide the strongest evidence.

Clinical Pearl: Clinical guidelines are often based on systematic reviews.

MCQ 58

A physician discusses treatment options with a patient, explains benefits and risks, and incorporates the patient's preferences into the final decision. This process is known as:

A. Polypharmacy

B. Shared decision-making

C. Therapeutic duplication

D. Pharmacovigilance

Answer: B

Explanation: Shared decision-making combines clinical evidence with patient values and preferences to select the most appropriate treatment.

Clinical Pearl: Shared decision-making improves adherence and patient satisfaction.

MCQ 59

Which of the following best describes pharmacovigilance?

A. Manufacturing pharmaceutical products

B. Monitoring, detecting, assessing, and preventing adverse drug reactions after drug marketing

C. Measuring drug potency

D. Calculating drug doses

Answer: B

Explanation: Pharmacovigilance focuses on the ongoing monitoring of medication safety throughout a drug's lifecycle.

Clinical Pearl: Reporting suspected adverse drug reactions contributes to safer medication use worldwide.

MCQ 60

A clinician reviews the patient's diagnosis, medical history, kidney function, current medications, allergies, and current clinical guidelines before prescribing therapy. Which principle is being applied?

A. Empirical prescribing

B. Evidence-based and rational pharmacotherapy

C. Polypharmacy

D. Defensive medicine

Answer: B

Explanation: Rational and evidence-based pharmacotherapy integrates clinical evidence with patient-specific factors to select the safest and most effective treatment.

Clinical Pearl: The best prescription is one that is evidence-based, individualized, effective, safe, and acceptable to the patient.

MCQ 61

Which route of drug administration is most appropriate for a patient who is unconscious but has stable circulation?

A. Oral

B. Sublingual

C. Intravenous

D. Topical

Answer: C

Explanation: An unconscious patient cannot safely swallow medications. Intravenous administration provides rapid and reliable drug delivery.

Clinical Pearl: Always assess airway, breathing, and circulation before selecting the route of drug administration.

MCQ 62

A drug that binds to a receptor without activating it and prevents an agonist from binding is called a(n):

A. Full agonist

B. Partial agonist

C. Competitive antagonist

D. Inverse agonist

Answer: C

Explanation: Competitive antagonists bind reversibly to receptors without activating them and compete with agonists for receptor binding.

Clinical Pearl: Increasing the agonist concentration can usually overcome competitive antagonism.

MCQ 63

Which statement regarding efficacy and potency is correct?

A. Potency is more clinically important than efficacy.

B. Efficacy is the maximum response a drug can produce.

C. Potency measures the safety of a drug.

D. Efficacy and potency are always directly proportional.

Answer: B

Explanation: Efficacy refers to the maximum therapeutic effect, whereas potency refers to the amount of drug required to produce a given effect.

Clinical Pearl: When choosing between drugs, efficacy is often more important than potency.

MCQ 64

A patient accidentally receives ten times the prescribed dose of insulin because of a decimal point error. This is an example of:

A. Type B adverse drug reaction

B. Medication error

C. Drug allergy

D. Drug intolerance

Answer: B

Explanation: Incorrect dosing caused by prescribing or administration mistakes is classified as a medication error.

Clinical Pearl: Always avoid trailing zeros (e.g., write 5 mg, not 5.0 mg).

MCQ 65

Which of the following patients is at the greatest risk for medication errors?

A. A healthy young adult taking one medication

B. A hospitalized older adult receiving multiple medications

C. A teenager using topical acne cream

D. An athlete taking vitamin supplements

Answer: B

Explanation: Older hospitalized patients with polypharmacy have a significantly higher risk of medication errors.

Clinical Pearl: Medication reconciliation is especially important in these patients.

MCQ 66

Which statement best describes a high-alert medication?

A. It is available only by prescription.

B. It has a high potential to cause serious patient harm if used incorrectly.

C. It is always expensive.

D. It has no generic equivalent.

Answer: B

Explanation: High-alert medications carry an increased risk of causing significant harm when errors occur.

Clinical Pearl: Examples include insulin, warfarin, heparin, opioids, and concentrated potassium chloride.

MCQ 67

Which of the following best illustrates rational drug use?

A. Prescribing antibiotics for every sore throat

B. Prescribing based on pharmaceutical advertisements

C. Choosing evidence-based therapy appropriate for the patient's diagnosis

D. Prescribing multiple drugs without reviewing current medications

Answer: C

Explanation: Rational drug use emphasizes evidence-based, individualized, and cost-effective therapy.

Clinical Pearl: Not every infection requires an antibiotic.

MCQ 68

Which statement regarding essential medicines is TRUE?

A. They are only used in developing countries.

B. They are selected solely because they are inexpensive.

C. They address the priority healthcare needs of the population.

D. They include only antibiotics.

Answer: C

Explanation: Essential medicines are selected based on public health relevance, efficacy, safety, quality, and cost-effectiveness.

Clinical Pearl: Every country may adapt the WHO Model List according to local healthcare needs.

MCQ 69

Which pharmacokinetic process primarily determines how a drug leaves the body?

A. Absorption

B. Distribution

C. Elimination

D. Receptor binding

Answer: C

Explanation: Elimination consists mainly of metabolism and excretion, removing drugs from the body.

Clinical Pearl: Renal and hepatic function strongly influence drug elimination.

MCQ 70

A patient reports taking an over-the-counter herbal supplement while receiving prescription medications. The clinician should primarily consider the possibility of:

A. Increased receptor selectivity

B. Drug interactions

C. Increased bioavailability of all drugs

D. Reduced drug potency only

Answer: B

Explanation: Herbal products may interact with prescription medications by altering drug metabolism or pharmacodynamic effects.

Clinical Pearl: Always ask patients about herbal products and dietary supplements.

MCQ 71

Which of the following is the best example of a narrow therapeutic index drug?

A. Vitamin C

B. Digoxin

C. Amoxicillin

D. Cetirizine

Answer: B

Explanation: Digoxin has a narrow margin between therapeutic and toxic concentrations.

Clinical Pearl: Therapeutic drug monitoring is recommended for several narrow therapeutic index drugs.

MCQ 72

The primary goal of pharmacovigilance is to:

A. Increase drug sales

B. Identify and reduce medication-related risks

C. Develop new dosage forms

D. Replace clinical trials

Answer: B

Explanation: Pharmacovigilance monitors medication safety after marketing and helps detect rare or delayed adverse effects.

Clinical Pearl: Reporting adverse drug reactions improves patient safety worldwide.

MCQ 73

Which healthcare professional is primarily responsible for verifying prescriptions, identifying drug interactions, and counseling patients?

A. Pharmacist

B. Radiologist

C. Physiotherapist

D. Laboratory technologist

Answer: A

Explanation: Pharmacists play a central role in ensuring safe and effective medication use.

Clinical Pearl: Effective collaboration between physicians, pharmacists, and nurses improves medication safety.

MCQ 74

Which factor should always be considered before prescribing a medication primarily eliminated by the kidneys?

A. Hair color

B. Renal function

C. Eye color

D. Blood type

Answer: B

Explanation: Impaired renal function may lead to drug accumulation and toxicity if doses are not adjusted.

Clinical Pearl: Serum creatinine and estimated glomerular filtration rate (eGFR) are commonly used to assess kidney function.

MCQ 75

A patient develops severe hypotension immediately after receiving the first dose of a medication because of a known pharmacological effect. This reaction is most likely classified as:

A. Type A adverse drug reaction

B. Type B adverse drug reaction

C. Type D adverse drug reaction

D. Type F adverse drug reaction

Answer: A

Explanation: Type A reactions are predictable and related to the known pharmacological action of the drug.

Clinical Pearl: Most adverse drug reactions encountered in clinical practice are Type A.

MCQ 76

Which statement best describes shared decision-making?

A. The physician alone selects the treatment.

B. The patient alone decides the treatment.

C. The clinician and patient work together using evidence and patient preferences.

D. Treatment is determined solely by hospital policy.

Answer: C

Explanation: Shared decision-making integrates clinical evidence with patient values and preferences.

Clinical Pearl: Shared decision-making improves adherence and patient satisfaction.

MCQ 77

Which of the following is considered the highest level of evidence when developing clinical practice guidelines?

A. Expert opinion

B. Case reports

C. Cohort studies

D. Systematic reviews and meta-analyses

Answer: D

Explanation: Systematic reviews and meta-analyses summarize evidence from multiple high-quality studies and provide the strongest support for clinical recommendations.

Clinical Pearl: Guidelines should be regularly updated as new evidence becomes available.

MCQ 78

The use of computerized provider order entry (CPOE) primarily helps reduce:

A. Drug manufacturing costs

B. Prescribing errors

C. Drug metabolism

D. Drug potency

Answer: B

Explanation: CPOE reduces errors caused by illegible handwriting, incomplete prescriptions, and transcription mistakes.

Clinical Pearl: Combining CPOE with clinical decision support systems further improves medication safety.

MCQ 79

Which patient counseling point is MOST important when prescribing a new medication?

A. Explain only the medication cost.

B. Explain the purpose of the medication, how to take it, possible adverse effects, and when to seek medical attention.

C. Tell the patient only the drug name.

D. Advise the patient to stop the medication if symptoms improve immediately.

Answer: B

Explanation: Comprehensive patient education improves adherence, therapeutic outcomes, and medication safety.

Clinical Pearl: Encourage patients to ask questions and report adverse effects promptly.

MCQ 80

A physician prescribes medication after reviewing current clinical guidelines, considering the patient's kidney function, allergies, concurrent medications, treatment goals, and personal preferences. This is the BEST example of:

A. Empirical prescribing

B. Polypharmacy

C. Evidence-based, patient-centered pharmacotherapy

D. Defensive medicine

Answer: C

Explanation: Evidence-based, patient-centered pharmacotherapy combines high-quality scientific evidence with clinical expertise and individual patient factors to optimize treatment outcomes.

Clinical Pearl: Safe prescribing requires balancing efficacy, safety, patient values, and cost-

effectiveness while continuously monitoringtherapeutic response.

MCQ 81

Which of the following best describes the primary goal of pharmacotherapy?

A. Eliminate all adverse drug reactions

B. Achieve the desired therapeutic effect with minimal toxicity

C. Prescribe the newest available medication

D. Use the highest possible drug dose

Answer: B

Explanation: The goal of pharmacotherapy is to maximize therapeutic benefit while minimizing adverse effects and toxicity.

Clinical Pearl: Always weigh the benefits of treatment against its potential risks.

MCQ 82

A physician prescribes a medication using its generic name rather than its brand name. The main advantage is that it:

A. Guarantees faster drug absorption

B. Reduces medication costs and prescribing errors

C. Increases drug potency

D. Eliminates adverse drug reactions

Answer: B

Explanation: Prescribing by generic name promotes rational prescribing, improves communication, and usually reduces healthcare costs.

Clinical Pearl: Approved generic drugs are therapeutically equivalent to their brand-name counterparts.

MCQ 83

Which patient is most likely to require individualized dose adjustment?

A. A healthy 25-year-old adult

B. A patient with chronic kidney disease

C. A patient with seasonal allergic rhinitis

D. A healthy adolescent

Answer: B

Explanation: Renal impairment decreases the elimination of many medications, increasing the risk of toxicity.

Clinical Pearl: Always assess renal function before prescribing renally excreted drugs.

MCQ 84

Which statement about adverse drug reactions (ADRs) is correct?

A. All ADRs are preventable.

B. Type A reactions are unpredictable.

C. Type A reactions are usually dose dependent and predictable.

D. Type B reactions account for most ADRs.

Answer: C

Explanation: Type A reactions are related to the known pharmacological effects of the drug and are usually predictable and dose dependent.

Clinical Pearl: Approximately 70–80% of ADRs are Type A reactions.

MCQ 85

Which of the following is an example of a medication error?

A. A patient develops a penicillin allergy.

B. A nurse administers medication to the wrong patient.

C. A patient develops nausea after chemotherapy.

D. A patient experiences an expected adverse effect of morphine.

Answer: B

Explanation: Administering medication to the wrong patient is a preventable medication error.

Clinical Pearl: Use at least two patient identifiers before administering medications.

MCQ 86

The WHO Model List of Essential Medicines is primarily intended to:

A. Replace national treatment guidelines.

B. Guide countries in selecting priority medicines.

C. Approve new drugs for marketing.

D. Regulate pharmaceutical prices.

Answer: B

Explanation: The WHO Model List serves as a reference for countries developing their National Essential Medicines Lists.

Clinical Pearl: Essential medicines improve access to safe, effective, and affordable treatment.

MCQ 87

Which statement regarding generic drugs is FALSE?

A. They contain the same active ingredient as the reference drug.

B. They must demonstrate bioequivalence.

C. They usually cost less than brand-name drugs.

D. They require different therapeutic doses than brand-name drugs.

Answer: D

Explanation: Generic drugs contain the same active ingredient and therapeutic dose as the corresponding brand-name product.

Clinical Pearl: Differences in tablet color or shape do not usually affect therapeutic outcomes.

MCQ 88

Which principle is fundamental to rational drug use?

A. Prescribe antibiotics for all respiratory infections.

B. Prescribe medications based on scientific evidence and patient needs.

C. Always prescribe multiple medications.

D. Use brand-name drugs whenever available.

Answer: B

Explanation: Rational drug use involves selecting the most appropriate medication based on evidence, patient characteristics, safety, and cost.

Clinical Pearl: Rational prescribing reduces medication errors and unnecessary healthcare costs.

MCQ 89

The PICO format is used to:

A. Classify adverse drug reactions.

B. Evaluate medication errors.

C. Develop focused clinical questions for evidence-based practice.

D. Measure therapeutic index.

Answer: C

Explanation: PICO stands for Patient (Problem), Intervention, Comparison, and Outcome and is used to formulate answerable clinical questions.

Clinical Pearl: A well-constructed PICO question improves literature searching and clinical decision-making.

MCQ 90

Which source provides the strongest evidence for selecting drug therapy?

A. Expert opinion

B. Case report

C. Randomized controlled trial

D. Systematic review and meta-analysis

Answer: D

Explanation: Systematic reviews and meta-analyses combine results from multiple high-quality studies and provide the highest level of evidence for therapeutic interventions.

Clinical Pearl: Evidence-based guidelines are commonly based on systematic reviews.

MCQ 91

A patient taking five different prescription medications is an example of:

A. Therapeutic duplication

B. Polypharmacy

C. Drug intolerance

D. Pharmacovigilance

Answer: B

Explanation: Polypharmacy is commonly defined as the concurrent use of five or more medications.

Clinical Pearl: Polypharmacy increases the risk of drug interactions and adverse drug reactions.

MCQ 92

Which healthcare professional is primarily responsible for educating patients about the safe use of prescribed medications at the time of dispensing?

A. Pharmacist

B. Radiographer

C. Pathologist

D. Physiotherapist

Answer: A

Explanation: Pharmacists play an important role in medication counseling, identifying interactions, and improving medication adherence.

Clinical Pearl: Effective counseling reduces medication errors and improves therapeutic outcomes.

MCQ 93

Which statement regarding medication reconciliation is correct?

A. It is performed only at hospital discharge.

B. It helps prevent medication omissions, duplications, and interactions.

C. It is unnecessary for outpatients.

D. It replaces patient counseling.

Answer: B

Explanation: Medication reconciliation compares a patient's medication list during transitions of care to reduce medication-related problems.

Clinical Pearl: Reconciliation should be performed at admission, transfer, and discharge.

MCQ 94

A physician carefully reviews current clinical guidelines before selecting therapy. This practice reflects:

A. Defensive medicine

B. Evidence-based pharmacotherapy

C. Empirical treatment only

D. Therapeutic duplication

Answer: B

Explanation: Evidence-based pharmacotherapy integrates current scientific evidence, clinical expertise, and patient preferences.

Clinical Pearl: Clinical guidelines support—but do not replace—clinical judgment.

MCQ 95

Which statement best describes shared decision-making?

A. The physician alone determines treatment.

B. The patient alone determines treatment.

C. Treatment decisions are made collaboratively using evidence and patient preferences.

D. Treatment is based only on medication cost.

Answer: C

Explanation: Shared decision-making promotes patient-centered care and improves adherence.

Clinical Pearl: Patients who understand their treatment plan are more likely to follow it.

MCQ 96

Which of the following is an important responsibility of pharmacovigilance programs?

A. Manufacturing medications

B. Detecting rare adverse drug reactions after marketing

C. Marketing pharmaceutical products

D. Determining drug prices

Answer: B

Explanation: Pharmacovigilance identifies rare and long-term adverse effects that may not have been detected during clinical trials.

Clinical Pearl: Reporting suspected ADRs contributes to safer medication use.

MCQ 97

A clinician prescribes the lowest effective dose of a medication to minimize toxicity. Which pharmacological principle is being applied?

A. Irrational prescribing

B. Rational drug use

C. Polypharmacy

D. Therapeutic duplication

Answer: B

Explanation: Using the lowest effective dose reduces the risk of adverse effects while maintaining therapeutic benefit.

Clinical Pearl: "Start low and go slow" is especially important in older adults.

MCQ 98

Which factor should be considered before prescribing any medication?

A. Patient allergies

B. Kidney and liver function

C. Current medications

D. All of the above

Answer: D

Explanation: Safe prescribing requires a comprehensive assessment, including allergies, organ function, concurrent medications, and comorbidities.

Clinical Pearl: A complete medication history helps prevent adverse drug reactions and interactions.

MCQ 99

A patient experiences an unexpected severe allergic reaction after the first dose of a medication despite appropriate prescribing. This event is best classified as:

A. Medication error

B. Type B adverse drug reaction

C. Type A adverse drug reaction

D. Therapeutic failure

Answer: B

Explanation: Type B (Bizarre) reactions are unpredictable, not dose dependent, and often immune-mediated.

Clinical Pearl: Penicillin-induced anaphylaxis is a classic Type B ADR.

MCQ 100

Which statement best summarizes the principles of modern pharmacology?

A. Prescribe the newest medication available regardless of cost.

B. Use multiple medications whenever possible.

C. Select evidence-based, safe, effective, patient-centered therapy while monitoring therapeutic response and adverse effects.

D. Avoid generic medications whenever possible.

Answer: C

Explanation: Modern pharmacology emphasizes rational prescribing, evidence-based medicine, patient safety, individualized therapy, and continuous monitoring to optimize therapeutic outcomes.

Clinical Pearl: The ideal prescription is effective, safe, individualized, evidence-based, affordable, and supported by patient education and follow-up.

End of Part I – General Principles of Pharmacology

Total Questions: 100
Format: Single Best Answer (SBA)
Coverage: All core principles of basic pharmacology, including drug nomenclature, classification, pharmacodynamics, adverse drug reactions, medication safety, rational prescribing, essential medicines, generic drugs, and evidence-based pharmacotherapy.

This completes Part I – General Principles of Pharmacology MCQs (Questions 1–100)

1. References
2. Brunton LL, Hilal-Dandan R, Knollmann BC, editors. Goodman & Gilman's The Pharmacological Basis of Therapeutics. 14th ed. New York, NY: McGraw Hill; 2023.
3. Katzung BG, Vanderah TW. Basic & Clinical Pharmacology. 16th ed. New York, NY: McGraw Hill; 2024.
4. Ritter JM, Flower RJ, Henderson G, Loke YK, MacEwan DJ, Rang HP. Rang & Dale's Pharmacology. 10th ed. Elsevier; 2024.
5. Whalen K. Lippincott Illustrated Reviews: Pharmacology. 8th ed. Philadelphia, PA: Wolters Kluwer; 2022.
6. Neal MJ. Medical Pharmacology at a Glance. 9th ed. Wiley-Blackwell; 2020.
7. Trevor AJ, Katzung BG, Kruidering-Hall M. Katzung & Trevor's Pharmacology: Examination & Board Review. 13th ed. McGraw Hill; 2021.
8. Ritter JM, Flower RJ, Henderson G, Loke YK. Rang & Dale's Pharmacology: Flashcards. Elsevier; latest available edition.
9. Katzung BG. Basic and Clinical Pharmacology: Study Guide and Review. McGraw Hill; latest available edition.
10. World Health Organization. WHO Model Formulary. Geneva: World Health Organization.
11. World Health Organization. Guide to Good Prescribing: A Practical Manual. Geneva: World Health Organization.
12. U.S. Food and Drug Administration. Drugs@FDA: FDA-Approved Drugs. U.S. Food and Drug Administration.
13. U.S. Food and Drug Administration. FDA Drug Safety Communications. U.S. Food and Drug Administration.
14. U.S. National Library of Medicine. DailyMed: Current Medication Information. National Library of Medicine.
15. Joint Formulary Committee. British National Formulary (BNF). London: BMJ Group and Pharmaceutical Press; latest available edition.
16. Brunton LL, Knollmann BC, editors. Goodman & Gilman's Manual of Pharmacology and Therapeutics. McGraw Hill.
17. Bertram G. Katzung. Basic & Clinical Pharmacology. Sections on pharmacokinetics, pharmacodynamics, drug receptors, drug metabolism, drug interactions, and adverse drug reactions. McGraw Hill.
18. Hall JE. Guyton and Hall Textbook of Medical Physiology. Elsevier. Sections relating to autonomic regulation, receptors, membrane transport, and physiological responses to drugs.
19. Jameson JL, Fauci AS, Kasper DL, Hauser SL, Longo DL, Loscalzo J, editors. Harrison's Principles of Internal Medicine. McGraw Hill. Relevant sections on clinical pharmacology and therapeutic drug use.
20. Katzung BG, Trevor AJ. Pharmacology Examination & Board Review. McGraw Hill. Questions and review material relevant to pharmacological principles and examination preparation.
21. International Council for Harmonisation of Technical Requirements for Pharmaceuticals for Human Use (ICH). ICH Harmonised Guidelines. Relevant guidance concerning clinical safety, pharmacokinetics, and drug development.
22. Recommended Online References
23. U.S. Food and Drug Administration (FDA). Drugs and Drug Safety.
24. National Library of Medicine (NLM). DailyMed.
25. National Library of Medicine. PubMed. Biomedical literature database.
26. World Health Organization (WHO). Medicines and Health Products.
27. European Medicines Agency (EMA). Medicines and safety information.
28. Note: Drug information, prescribing recommendations, and regulatory information should be checked against the most current official sources because drug labeling, safety warnings, and clinical recommendations may change over time.